I0134917

Vitamin D Deficiency and Autoimmune Disease

Vitamin D Deficiency and Autoimmune Disease

How Vitamin D Prevents Autoimmune Disease

Wayne Persky

Persky Farms

United States

First published and distributed in the United States of America by:
Persky Farms, 19242 Darrs Creek Rd, Bartlett, TX 76511-4022. Tel.: (1)254-718-1125; Fax: (1)254-527-3682. www.perskyfarms.com

Copyright: This book is protected under the US Copyright Act of 1976, as amended, and all other applicable international, federal, state, and local laws. All rights reserved. No part of this book may be reproduced by any mechanical, photographic, or electronic process, or in the form of an audio recording, nor may it be transmitted or otherwise copied for public or private use, other than the "fair use" purposes allowed by copyright law, without prior or written permission of the publisher.

Disclaimer and Legal Notice: The information contained in this book is intended solely for general educational purposes, and is not intended, nor implied, to be a substitute for professional medical advice relative to any specific medical condition or question. The advice of a physician or other health care provider should always be sought for any questions regarding any medical condition. Specific diagnoses and therapies can only be provided by the reader's physician. The author and the publisher specifically disclaim any and all liability arising directly or indirectly from the use or application of any information contained in this book.

Please note that much of the information in this book is based on personal experience and anecdotal evidence. Although the author and publisher have made every reasonable attempt to achieve complete accuracy of the content, they assume no responsibility for errors or omissions. If you should choose to use any of this information, use it according to your best judgment, and at your own risk. Because your particular situation will not exactly match the examples upon which this information is based, you should adjust your use of the information and recommendations to fit your own personal situation.

This book does not recommend or endorse any specific tests, products, procedures, opinions, or other information that may be mentioned anywhere in the book. This information is provided for educational purposes, and reliance on any tests, products, procedures, or opinions mentioned in the book is solely at the reader's own risk. Any trademarks, service marks, product names, or named features are assumed to be the property of their respective owners, and are used only for reference. There is no implied endorsement when these terms are used in this book.

Copyright © Wayne Persky, 2013. All rights reserved worldwide.

ISBN 978-1-7328220-3-0

Table of Contents

Introduction

Vitamin D has become a much-discussed topic in recent years. Some medical authorities claim that vitamin D deficiency is a widespread problem these days. Furthermore, they argue that official government and medical association published guidelines for safe vitamin D levels are inadequate. Many insist that those levels should be substantially higher, in order to offer better protection against the risk of disease development. As additional research articles are published, more and more of them show an association between vitamin D deficiency and many common diseases.

Other medical and government-affiliated authorities insist that such claims are groundless, and the problem is way overblown. Who is right? Can we afford to ignore the problem while medical professionals and government advisory panels argue about it? Or does waiting for the experts to settle their disagreements amount to playing Russian roulette with our health? Reading this book should provide the information you need to form your own informed opinion, so that you can answer those questions to your own satisfaction

It's generally agreed that vitamin D supports our overall health in many ways. This has been documented by numerous research articles that verify many of the details of how this occurs. Vitamin D appears to support our health primarily by enhancing certain aspects of our immune system, in order to improve the

Introduction

ability of the immune system to prevent disease and to destroy pathogens or malignant cells that are associated with existing disease. It has been well established that vitamin D deficiency is associated with the development of many chronic, difficult-to-treat diseases, such as inflammatory bowel disease (IBD), for example.

Research shows that not only does a vitamin D deficiency create an environment favorable to the development of IBD, but the existence of an IBD tends to deplete the body's available supply of vitamin D. This creates a self-perpetuating problem that prevents our immune system from being able to resolve the symptoms, without medical intervention. For medical research references that support these statements, see chapter 1 and refer to the respective numbered references listed for each chapter in the back of the book.

As you read this book, you will learn why IBDs are able to deplete our vitamin D level. And you will learn why maintaining an adequate vitamin D level in our bloodstream may be the most important thing we can do to prevent the development of inflammatory bowel disease (or some other autoimmune disease).

Furthermore, research suggests that by similar mechanisms, low vitamin D levels appear to be implicated in the development of virtually all other autoimmune diseases as well. So just what are the unique attributes of vitamin D that enable it to provide such powerful benefits for enhancing our ability to fight disease?

Introduction

Until very recently, we could only guess, but recent research has shed a significant amount of light on this mystery, and these discoveries allow us to understand many of the details of how this may happen. In this book we will explore the details of how a vitamin D deficiency creates an environment that promotes autoimmune disease. And more importantly, we will gain valuable insight into how and why maintaining a sufficiently high blood level of vitamin D appears to be the key to proper immune system functioning, so that opportunities for the development of autoimmune disease are greatly reduced.

Vitamin D possesses many health benefits, far too many to explore in detail in a single book. So in this book we will primarily focus on the unique powers that vitamin D conveys to the immune system. We're especially interested in the specific ways that vitamin D is able to activate certain aspects of the immune system that enable it to prevent the development and perpetuation of autoimmune disease. But along the way, we'll briefly discuss some of the other diseases that have been found to be associated with vitamin D deficiency. This supporting information will help us to understand how extensively vitamin D is integrated into the proper functioning of our immune system. Research data clearly indicate that without an adequate supply of vitamin D, our immune system quickly becomes severely crippled.

In the United States, vitamin D blood levels are listed in nanograms per milliliter (ng/ml). For the convenience of readers who live in countries where vitamin D is measured in international units, in this book those vitamin D levels will be followed

Introduction

by the equivalent number in nanomoles per liter (nmol/l), enclosed in parentheses.

Please note that although this book may be relatively short, parts of it are packed with important information that should be very carefully read. In order to fully understand the implications of some of the research results that are cited, it may be necessary to read the information and then carefully re-read it, possibly more than once, in some instances.

Research articles that are referenced within the text of the chapters of this book are designated according to "DOI" identifiers (whenever DOI identifiers have been assigned to the articles). For anyone not familiar with the use of DOI designations, DOI stands for "Digital Object Identifier", and a DOI is a unique alphanumeric string authorized by the International DOI Foundation, and assigned by the publisher, to identify digital documents, and provide a permanent link to their respective locations on the Internet. In order to locate an article, entering the listed DOI identifier into any search engine, should lead to a link to the article. Research articles that have not been assigned a DOI identifier are designated by a conventional Internet Uniform Resource Identifier (URL) that can be used to access the article on the Internet.

Chapter 1

How Autoimmune Disease Develops

What exactly is autoimmune disease?

The formal medical requirements that must be met in order for a disease to be classified as autoimmune are necessarily rigid. Most of us would consider them to be not only boring, but rather mysterously-worded, reminding us somewhat of a riddle.

Researchers Rosea and Bona, (1994) postulated the formal medical conditions that must be met in order for a syndrome to be classified as an autoimmune disease. These requirements stipulate that an autoimmune disease must be characterized by:[1]

1. Direct evidence of the transfer of pathogenic antibodies or pathogenic T-cells

2. Indirect evidence based on reproduction of the autoimmune disease in experimental animals

3. Circumstantial evidence from clinical clues

In simple language, for a disease to qualify as autoimmune, it must provoke the immune system to produce either antibodies that trigger subsequent inflammatory immune system actions, or killer T-cells, or both, and the target of these actions must be the body's own cells. That is to say, the immune system response to the disease must result in damage to "self" (the body's own tissue). Obviously this is not a literal translation of the medical descripton of autoimmune disease, but I believe that it portrays autoimmunity more clearly, so that we can better understand how it relates to the subject matter in this book.

What causes autoimmune disease, and hows does it begin?

At one time we thought that the reason why some people developed autoimmune diseases while others did not, was mostly a matter of luck — bad luck. We mostly blamed it on our genes. If we happened to inherit certain "disease-prone" genes from our parents, then we feared the worst, while hoping for the best. If one or both of our parents had rheumatoid arthritis for example, we could literally see the handwriting on the wall, regarding our own future.

Everything happens for a reason.

And the state of our health is no exception. The reasons are not always obvious, and they are not always due to the factors that we have been led to believe are responsible. It seems that researchers are discovering that many beliefs long upheld as facts by mainstream medicine, are not actually proven facts at all, especially in the area of diet and its effects on long-term health.

Many of these mistakes were made decades or even centuries ago, when incorrect assumptions were made, typically based on faulty science. A prime example of a mistaken medical policy based on faulty science can be found in one that was actually mandated by politics. In the 1970s, animal fat and cholesterol in the diet were declared by the USDA to be our "number 1 public health problem".[2] This convoluted turn of events took place after the chairman of a senate committee that had been appointed to modernize USDA diet recommendations chose to allow a staff member who did not have a scientific background, to write the new policy, and in doing so he chose to adopt faulty health research data instead of valid research data. So much for allowing politicians to dictate diet and health advice.

That mistake is still in the process of being corrected. In other cases, mistaken claims were made due to incorrect conclusions based on "cherry picking" of data resulting from research projects, or simply invalid conclusions based on confounded (invalid) research data. And after the claims were repeated for decades, it's not surprising that most medical professionals assumed that they were proven facts.

As is the case with most science-based disciplines, in medicine, once a concept is accepted as a proven fact, it's not likely that the status will be changed, without a Herculean effort. It can take decades, and mountains of research data to eventually bring about a correction of a long-standing mistake. And sadly, it seems that there have been a disproportional number of mistakes made regarding accepted medical advice relating to the effects of diet on health.

Today we know that obesity is not caused by eating animal fat. It's caused by eating excessive amounts of carbohydrates, primarily grains and sugars. Farmers, ranchers, and feedlot operators have always known that. When they want to fatten feedlot cattle, hogs, or lambs as quickly as possible, they don't feed them fat — they feed them grain, a lot of grain. And today we are finally once again realizing something that our ancestors have always known — namely, that eating animal fat is beneficial for health (not the other way around).

Likewise, we now know that cholesterol in the diet is not simply absorbed unchanged (as cholesterol) and added to existing cholesterol in the body. Rather, like all foods, it's broken down by the digestive system into individual amino acids, and used by the body as building blocks, along with other nutrients, to make new cells. We are relearning that heredity and lifestyle choices primarily determine our cholesterol level, while cholesterol in the diet has only a very limited effect.

This problem with lapses in the reliability of mainstream diet and health advice can probably be attributed to the fact that medical school training typically provides only the most rudimentary amount of education in nutrition and dietary considerations for health. And physicians are not likely to be exposed to nutritional or dietary training on the job, either, because just as is the case in med school, most of their on-the-job training revolves around treatment by the use of prescription drugs.

"Diet" is typically viewed as something that is utilized for weight loss. Most doctors do not seem to view diet as a practical way to treat disease, or other health issues (other than obesity and celiac disease). And of course because of the lack of adequate training of physicians by medical schools, it seems that most of our diet and health advice and guidelines come from government agencies or advertising claims made by food processors. So it's not surprising that so many of us feel that much of our food supply seems to be becoming more unhealthy with each passing year

Genes play a huge role in our health.
But we also know that much more is involved. Thanks to recent advances in research, we are learning how certain environmental factors determine how our genes affect our future health, and most importantly, we are beginning to understand how those factors may affect our susceptibility to disease. We are learning that we have the power to do something that we have long yearned for, but never realized that we already possess — namely the power to manipulate those genes to our advantage.

In this book we will learn how autoimmune disease begins and how it develops. And we will explore ways to take advantage of certain powers built into our immune system that can enable us to improve our chances of preventing those diseases from developing. But first we need to consider some background information to use as a platform for advancing our understanding of our immune system and how autoimmune disease begins.

There are currently many diseases that are categorized as autoimmune.

The term "autoimmune" is used to describe a reaction by the immune system that is directed against "self". That is to say, an autoimmune disease is defined as a syndrome in which the immune system engages in behavior that results in damage to tissue that is part of its own body.

No widely-accepted official medical position exists.

No one has ever conclusively proven how diseases labeled as autoimmune actually develop (at least not as of the date of this writing), so it appears that there is no established official opinion on this issue. Researchers have observed that certain conditions are associated with the development of autoimmune disease, and it seems likely that at least some of these conditions may be a prerequisite for all types of autoimmune disease. Over the years, many researchers have offered suggestions or theories (without proof) about how certain individual autoimmune diseases may develop.

But to date at least, no medical researcher has offered a fundamental analysis of the basic ingredients that actually lead up to the point where all the necessary conditions that predispose to autoimmune disease are met. And no one has been able to provide proof of a general sequence of events that might lead up to the point where the development of autoimmune disease is eminent.

A prominent researcher has offered a theory.

As an example of the current official medical thinking on this issue, consider the theory recently offered by a leading researcher in the field of celiac disease.[3] This particular theory suggests that three necessary conditions must exist in order for autoimmune disease to develop.

1. A corrupt association between the innate and the adaptive immune system responses must exist
2. The immune system must be exposed to exogenous (external to the body) antigens on a chronic basis

3. Certain predisposing genes must be present, and a state of increased intestinal permeability (also known as leaky gut) must exist

I don't fully agree with the first claim in that theory (the assumption that the immune system must become corrupt in order for an autoimmune-type disease to develop), because in my opinion the real-world circumstances of this phenomenon do not actually involve immune system corruption. As we shall see in chapter 5, the problem is actually due to an oversight, or lack of understanding, on our part.

Vitamin D Deficiency and Autoimmune Disease

While the observations in the researcher's theory (that are listed above) appear to be correct (with the personal reservation noted above), and they provide useful information, note that this description does not actually address the reasons why autoimmune disease tends to develop in the first place. Instead, it skips ahead and simply states the conditions necessary for the development of an autoimmune syndrome at a point in time where the actual onset of autoimmune disease may occur at any moment.

In other words, it does not tell us exactly what events in our life may lead up to the development of autoimmune disease, it merely tells us that if we happen to find ourselves in a position where these conditions are met, then we had better look out, because we are predisposed (at that moment in time) to the development of one or more autoimmune diseases. It's important, in my opinion, to recognize that if we allow ourselves to reach the point where those three conditions apply to us, then the development of autoimmune disease is very likely imminent. It's possible that we may have already reached a critical point where it may be too late to prevent autoimmune disease from being triggered, unless extraordinary preventative methods are applied.

So clearly, it seems prudent to take steps that might prevent us from reaching such a precipice where the development of an autoimmune syndrome might be imminent. But of course in order to do that, we need to understand more about how the immune system functions, and in particular, we need to understand the details of how and why it sometimes malfunctions.

In general, the mainstream medical community doesn't appear to have whole-heartedly adopted this relatively new theory yet at this point, and most practitioners seem to cling to older established principles. Rather than to treat autoimmune disease as a pattern of syndromes with a common etiology (similar cause or origin), most medical professionals seem to view each autoimmune disease individually, as though each autoimmune disease is unique, and exists independently of all others. That is to say, most autoimmune diseases are typically treated as though they are unrelated to other autoimmune diseases.

While it is true that some rheumatologists are beginning to recognize that certain autoimmune diseases are related, it appears that most physicians still tend to think of them separately, and more importantly, they typically prescribe a treatment regimen that deals with each one individually. Because of this simplified approach, in some situations medications prescribed for one disease may actually make the symptoms of another disease more severe. Or worse yet, some treatments may actually lead to the development of additional autoimmune diseases.

What if all types of autoimmune disease had a common origin?

What if the various autoimmune syndromes were not separate and unique issues, as they are typically viewed by many physicians? What if they all had a common origin? If this were the

Vitamin D Deficiency and Autoimmune Disease

case, then if we were to somehow find ourselves in a position where we were at a high risk of developing some form of autoimmune disease, it follows that our genetics might be likely to play an important role in determining which autoimmune disease (or diseases) would be the most likely to develop. And of course this seems to be exactly what happens in most cases.

But the more important question is, "Why would we be in a position where we are vulnerable to developing an autoimmune disease in the first place?" Most of us try to lead a healthy lifestyle. While we may not always eat an ideal diet, we usually don't go out of our way to eat foods that we know to be detrimental to good health. And while we may not always be able to get as much exercise as we would like, we try to remain active, and we try to exercise on at least a somewhat regular basis.

And it's worth noting that we are all aware of highly-trained and dedicated athletes who supposedly follow the best health advice available, but who develop the same autoimmune issues as the rest of us. So what has to go wrong in our life to cause us to end up in a situation where even though we are trying hard to do everything right, and we seem healthy, we suddenly find ourselves predisposed to developing an autoimmune type disease? Obviously, if we knew the answer to that we just might be able to prevent it from happening.

That question bothered me for years as I found myself battling several autoimmune issues of my own. I found it difficult to understand why I was suddenly dealing with not just one, but several such issues. After all, one of the conditions proclaimed by immune system experts to be a primary cause of allergies and autoimmune disease in modern society is the claim that we grow up "too sanitary" these days. But as we will see on the next page, that theory doesn't appear to apply to me.

Are we "too clean"?

Many experts believe that our society has grown to be so clean and so afraid of exposure to dirt (and everything that term implies) that our immune system is no longer adequately challenged as it is developing, while we are growing up. They believe that this causes our immune system to become bored (as if it has a mind of its own), and the absence of adequate challenges somehow causes it to become corrupt. And they believe that this inspires our immune system to begin to launch attacks against ordinary, or even non-existent foreign invaders, or against selected cells of our own body, presumably to relieve its own boredom. In either event, since no legitimate targets are present in such a scenario, attacks of this type can only damage the body's own tissue. If this type of behavior should continue to the point where it occurs regularly, the result would be the development of autoimmune disease.

I suppose this theory is intended to be a corollary of the old English proverb, "An idle brain is the devil's workshop". So those who promote this theory of immune system corruption are saying that an idle immune system becomes a corrupt immune system, simply because it becomes bored, and so it "chooses" to revolt against the system, and pursue its own fantasies (so to speak), just to remain occupied. Think about that for a moment.

Vitamin D Deficiency and Autoimmune Disease

Does that seem logical? Does it meet the standards of plain old common sense?

Could growing up under conditions that are "too sanitary" actually cause allergies to develop?

And conversely, does being exposed to plenty of immune system challenges while we are growing up help to prevent allergies? My own experience certainly doesn't suggest that the theory has much validity. At least it certainly didn't seem to work for me.

I grew up on what is now known as a family farm (back in those days it was simply an ordinary, everyday farm) in the 1940s and '50s. As a young child, I played in the dirt at every opportunity. which was virtually every day except when the weather was too cold, or it was raining, or something of that sort. Back in those days, before the concept of the family farm fell victum to government farm program policies designed to force farmers to get bigger or get out, most farms were populated with a wide variety of animals, because farm families produced most of the food that they ate. And they took the surplus eggs, milk, and butter to town on weekends, to trade for staples such as flour, salt, and pepper, and sometimes canned goods, and other items, if their fruit and vegetable supply from their own garden had become depleted.

The members of our family, together with help from our neighbors and relatives who lived nearby, processed our own pork and beef, and we even cured our own bacon and ham back in those days. And in return, we helped our neighbors whenever they needed to restock their meat supply. If fried chicken was on the menu for Sunday dinner after church, we usually took care of that little processing chore on Saturday.

Cattle, hogs, horses, mules, sheep, and goats roamed in fenced-in pastures, with access to barns, of course. But chickens, turkeys, ducks, geese, dogs, and cats usually roamed free in the farmyard, and they played (and did everything else that animals and birds do) in the same dirt in which I played. I can still remember the time when I was probably about 3 years old, that I passed what appeared to me to be a huge worm (probably Ascaris lumbricoides), after being given a vermicide by my mother. I can still remember how relieved my mother seemed to be, after she glanced in the pot and saw the evidence of success. So clearly, I had plenty of exposure to immune system stimulants while my immune system was in the developmental stage.

And yet I had asthma as a child, and one night when I was about 12 or 13, I had an attack that was unusually severe. Doctors still made house calls back in those days, and if the local small-town doctor had not been willing to come out to our house in the wee hours of the morning to give me a cortisone shot, I probably would not have lasted until sunrise. According to my parents and the doctor, I was beginning to turn blue from oxygen starvation. I can still remember how exhausted I felt the next day. I hurt all over from the extreme effort that had been required for so many hours, just to draw each breath.

Vitamin D Deficiency and Autoimmune Disease

As I entered my teens, the asthma seemed to fade away but it was replaced by an increasing allergy to pollen, resulting in classic hayfever symptoms. When I was in my 20s I suddenly found that I could no longer tolerate a popular brand of mouthwash that I had been using daily for years. One day within seconds after I put it in my mouth and began to swish it around, the lining of my mouth felt as though it were on fire. And after I spit the liquid out, all it took was a glance in the mirror to confirm that the lining of my mouth was bright red and clearly inflamed.

After that, my immune system issues seemed to hold steady until I reached my mid-50s. At that point the wheels began to fall off, as some of the early symptoms of gluten sensitivity began to show up. Of course it never dawned on me at the time, that something in my diet might be causing the symptoms, nor did any of my doctors ever make the connection. Things went steadily downhill from there, and eventually I found myself as sick as a dog (as we used to say out here in the country), with uncontrollable diarrhea, nausea, migraines, muscle and joint stiffness, and aches and pains, and even brain fog. And after subjecting me to every test he could think of, my GI specialist informed me there was nothing wrong with me. While he didn't go so far as to insist that I needed to see a psychiatrist, he did mention in passing that it might be helpful. That's when it dawned on me that I was on my own, because it was painfully obvious that help was not likely to be forthcoming through medical channels.

So much for the theory that kids need to play in the dirt, in order to avoid immune system problems.

Playing in the dirt obviously didn't work for me. And so much for the medical community's understanding of autoimmune type issues in general, and food sensitivities in particular. I did eventually manage to figure out on my own what was causing my symptoms (multiple food sensitivities associated with gluten sensitivity), and I was able to resolve my symptoms and get my life back, but that's another story that's not necessarily important to the subject of this book. If more information is desired, that story, and detailed information on food sensitivities, and how they are related to autoimmune diseases, can be found in the book *Microscopic Colitis* (Persky, 2012).[4]

So what really causes us to develop diseases claimed to be due to an "overactive" immune system?

Fast forward a few years to the point where, with the background that I have described in mind, I set out to find some answers. After spending many, many hours tracking down and studying hundreds and hundreds of research articles that have been published in medical journals, I was able to locate a surprising number of articles that offered important and illuminating clues. I discovered that when the findings of those research projects were considered together, they answered a lot of questions, and the data led to sort of an epiphany for me.

Vitamin D Deficiency and Autoimmune Disease

The evidence points to a combination of events in our lives that appears to explain how those previously-mentioned predisposing conditions might come about. That is to say, the research data suggest that a certain unique combination of issues in our personal environment can place us in a position where those conditions are satisfied, thereby making us candidates for the development of autoimmune disease. This theory is described in detail in chapter 16 of the previously-mentioned book, *Microscopic Colitis* (Persky, 2012).

Rather than to include a detailed description of the theory here, I will quote a brief summary of the theory from the book:

> *In a nutshell, chronic stress creates an environment where disease can develop. In that environment, mast cells become unstable, and existing food and drug sensitivities trigger mast cell responses that involve the release of modulators that generate the inflammation that leads to increased intestinal permeability, thereby providing the mechanism that leads to what is commonly considered to be an autoimmune-type process.*
>
> *But even if food or drug-sensitivities do not yet exist, stress can lead to the inappropriate degranulation of mast cells, causing an inflammatory environment, resulting in increased intestinal permeability. And once any of the genes that predispose to autoimmune disease are triggered, the genes that predispose to certain food sensitivities and drug-sensitivities, known to be associated with increased intestinal permeability, will also be triggered (as we learned in chapter seven). The resulting production of antibodies to food antigens will virtually*

guarantee that the stress produced by the clinical symptoms will lead to a self-perpetuating syndrome. Obviously, this adds up to be the immune system equivalent of a perfect storm. (pp. 220–221)

The term "degranulation" in the above quote refers to the release of proinflammatory granules contained within mast cells. Some of these agents (such as histamine) initiate inflammation directly, while others serve as messengers to trigger subsequent inflammatory responses from other components of the immune system.

You may have noticed that the quote refers to so-called "autoimmune-type" diseases or issues, rather than to simply refer to them as autoimmune diseases. There is a reason for the use of that particular terminology. And that reason can be summed up by another quote from the same chapter in the book (Persky, 2012).

According to my theory, autoimmune disease may not even exist

There is a possibility that the medical issues that the medical community chooses to categorize as autoimmune diseases may not actually be associated with autoimmune reactions at all. As we saw in chapters 8 and 9, our digestive system did not evolve to digest gluten, nor did it evolve to tolerate the various drugs that in so many individuals, seem to trigger what the medical community refers to as an autoimmune response. Though some drugs are derived from plants and other natural sources, most drugs available these days, and gluten, casein and soy, are foreign proteins, by definition (as far as our diges-

tive system is concerned), and our immune system is designed to keep foreign items out of our digestive system, out of our circulatory system, and out of our body, in general.

If we continue to ingest those items despite the fact that our body is desperately trying to tell us to avoid them, we shouldn't be surprised when we develop increased intestinal permeability. Nor should we be surprised if we eventually develop one or more so-called autoimmune diseases. We have to do our part, and stop flooding our digestive system with antigens. All that we have to do to stop the so-called autoimmune reaction is to stop ingesting those foreign items. If we do that, the reaction will fade away. And as long as we avoid ingesting those items in the future, additional reactions will not be triggered. So how could this process be considered to be a true autoimmune reaction if it can be stopped and subsequently prevented, by such a simple and logical process as eliminating the offending foods from our diet?

Obviously, if an exogenous agent (an ingested antigen) is responsible for triggering the reaction, then it's not an autoimmune reaction; it's just a normal immune system reaction — our body's way of trying to tell us to stop trying to poison ourselves with that stuff so that we can get on with our life. It's not rocket science; it's simply common sense. (pp. 225–226)

So it follows that if an autoimmune-type disease can be shown to be due to something that we are ingesting, or some material that we physically contact during our regular routine, then the official medical description of an autoimmune disease misses the point, and provides a misleading interpretation of the event. Why? Simply because this isn't an autoimmune reaction at all. Instead, it's simply an ordinary immune system response to something in our environment to which we have developed a sensitivity. If removing a food sensitivity from our diet, discontinuing the use of a drug, or avoiding contact with a material to which we are sensitive, can halt the symptoms, then obviously the immune system response can hardly be considered to be autoimmune. Clearly, in that situation, the primary reaction was initiated by an antigen outside the body. That, by definition, constitutes a normal immune system response, not an autoimmune response.

The problem is that diseases labeled as "Autoimmune" cannot be shown to be self-sustaining.

Medical experts base their justification for labeling such reactions as autoimmune, on the observation that antibodies can be found in the blood against certain normal body proteins (such as transglutaminase enzyme). While it is certainly true that anti-tissue transglutaminase antibodies can exist during such reactions, this is a moot point, since those antibody levels quickly fade away when the external antigens responsible for triggering the reaction are totally avoided.

If the reaction were truly autoimmune, it would be self-perpetuating, even in the absence of those exogenous antigens. Clearly, that does not happen, so how could the reactions be legitimately classified as autoimmune? Why would a secondary reaction that cannot occur in the absence of a primary reaction be considered to be legitimate on its own merits? Obviously most medical professionals will disagree with my viewpoint on this issue, but in essence it boils down to a matter of semantics.

However one chooses to view this issue, the bottom line is that if the external triggers are removed, then the so-called autoimmune reaction will fade away and it will not resume, unless the triggers are reintroduced. To my way of thinking, that does not describe a true autoimmune syndrome, because it is not actually self-perpetuating — it relies on an exogenous antigen to maintain the reaction, and the primary reaction is obviously the result of a legitimate immune system response. Therefore it appears that the official medical description of autoimmunity is flawed.

Summary

The current medical view of the cause of autoimmune disease is based on a theory that if the immune system is chronically exposed to external antigens, and if intestinal permeability is present, then the immune system somehow becomes corrupt, and begins to attack the body.

My own theory defines the specific details that actually lead up to that state, by describing the roles of chronic stress and mast cell degranulation, together with increased intestinal permeability, to result in an ordinary immune system reaction against an external antigen. And based on published, peer-reviewed medical research reports, it appears that chronic, inappropriate mast cell degranulation is virtually always involved in these reactions.

How Autoimmune Disease Develops

In contrast to the medical theory, there's some question in my mind about whether the assumption that the immune system must become corrupt in order for an autoimmune-type disease to develop is actually a legitimate point. I say this because as we will see in later chapters, the immune system corruption is actually a self-inflicted condition, due to our lack of providing the body with an adequate source of vitamin D. And it seems clear to me that the reaction described as "autoimmune" by the medical community is actually outside of the domain of a true autoimmune reaction by definition, since in most cases the reaction can be stopped at any time, simply by the avoidance of the external antigen that is responsible for triggering the immune system response.

Under those conditions, while there may indeed be collateral damage to the body's own tissue, and even the production of antibodies against a normal body enzyme, the primary immune system response is not directed against "self". Instead, it is clearly directed at one or more external antigens. This is verified by the way that the autoantibody levels quickly decline when the external antigens are avoided, thus proving that the reaction cannot be self-perpetuating in the absence of the external antigens.

Chapter 2

Conditions Necessary for Healing to Occur

Healing begins with inflammation.

Healing is the process by which damaged, diseased, or dead tissue is replaced with new, healthy tissue. Healing can occur by two different mechanisms.

1. Damaged cells can be replaced by new healthy cells in a regeneration process, so that the exact original configuration of the tissue is restored

2. The damaged issue can be repaired, and in this case it is replaced by scar tissue

The normal process of healing human tissue seems like a paradox at first glance.

It would seem logical that healing would begin with a calming, soothing process. But instead, healing begins with inflammation. During this initial stage of healing, the area becomes reddened, and tender, and swelling occurs as fluids accumulate in the tissues due to the leakage of serum from nearby blood vessels. In most cases, healing involves both of these methods (both replacement of some cells, and repair of others), especially in the healing of wounds.

The organs of the body are comprised of various types of tissue, and different types of tissue perform different functions. Regardless of its functional purpose, tissue is made up of individual cells, many of them having a specialized design, making them uniquely suitable for the job they are designed to do.

Cells are supported and held in place by either a basement membrane or a network of connective tissue (known as collagen). Normally when cells are damaged, the connective tissue is not destroyed and therefore it will still be functional even if the cells adjacent to it are dead. As long as the connective tissue is intact, cellular damage can be healed by regenerating new cells, identical to the original cells.

Before damaged cells can be replaced however, they must be removed, so they are marked by the immune system for destruction as part of the process of programmed cell death. This is the same mechanism used by the body for normal replacement of cells that are old and are scheduled for routine replacement on a

24

regular schedule. The medical term for programmed cell death is "apoptosis".

Certain cells cannot be healed simply by the regeneration of new cells to replace the damaged ones. They can only be healed by repair (which results in the formation of scar tissue). Such cells include muscles in the heart and neurons used by the central nervous system, or those used by the enteric nervous system (which controls the digestive system and communicates with the central nervous system). In any situation where the connective tissue network of collagen is damaged, such damage must be repaired, resulting in the creation of scar tissue.

If the damage is due to an incision or a wound, the first step in the healing process will be clot formation in order to stop the bleeding. While the loss of blood is typically viewed as undesirable, it is in fact very helpful for washing away pathogens to which the wound may have been exposed, such as bacteria, viruses, and fungi. The clot which forms to stop the bleeding is the next barrier which helps to prevent infectious agents from entering the body or the bloodstream. Lymphocytes (white blood cells) will then infiltrate into the injured tissue to initiate the inflammation process. In the case of a wound or incision, the lymphocytes will typically be neutrophils. These will be followed by macrophages and other cells that are sent by the immune system to clean up any remaining invaders that shouldn't be there (such as bacteria, viruses, and fungi). All of the resulting debris, including any remaining original dead or damaged cells, fluids, and any residues from the destruction of both damaged cells and pathogens, must be removed from the site in order for healing to proceed.

The matrix comprised of connective tissue (made of collagen) that holds all the cells together in the proper shape, contains fibroblasts, which are present in all connective tissue for the express purpose of maintaining and repairing collagen. Fibroblasts are special cells that contain all the raw materials needed to reconstruct the collagen-based matrix. Growth hormones and other chemicals are released during the debriding (cleanup) process, in order to encourage the fibroblasts to produce new collagen to fill the void left by an open wound. When the healing process is complete, a scar will mark the area where the repair was made.

Infection does not actually generate inflammation.

While we normally tend to think that inflammation is caused by an infection of some type, that's not really true. The inflammation is actually due to our body's response to the infection, as our immune system attempts to destroy the invaders, and this is a critical distinction. Normally this process works well. But if the inflammation fails to end the threat, then the inflammation will continue indefinitely and lead to unanticipated consequences — consequences that the immune system is not designed to handle.

Consider the intestinal inflammation associated with inflammatory bowel disease. With an IBD, cellular damage is not a simple discrete event. Instead, the propagation of new damage is perpetuated by the autoimmune process, so that at virtually any instant in time, new damage is continually being generated by the inflammatory reactions that are taking place. As long as new inflammation is being generated, there is always additional debris that needs to be removed. Therefore, the healing process effectively becomes stuck at the first stage, and cannot proceed, because the ongoing inflammatory process associated with an IBD results in a chronic cycle of damage.

Damage caused by inflammation in the intestines heals very slowly.

Even after the inflammation is stopped, healing of intestinal tissue takes much longer than would normally be expected when compared with the healing of other organs in the body.. I'm not aware of any research studies that have been done in an attempt to determine healing times associated with Crohn's disease or ulcerative colitis, but this has been done with celiac disease (which is actually an inflammatory bowel disease). With celiac disease, treatment consists of adopting a gluten-free diet. But even after a gluten-free diet is adopted and clinical symptoms disappear, physical healing of the cells in the mucosa of the small intestine actually progresses very, very slowly.

Kids heal much faster than adults.

Follow-up research shows that except in pediatric cases (kids heal much faster than adults), healing typically requires at least 3 to 5 years, or longer (in adults).[1,2] It's a fact of life that as we age we heal more slowly, unfortunately. And in some cases, the damage never completely heals. It's not known whether this is due to some degree of continuing inflammation resulting from a less-than-perfect diet, or whether the aging process results in a diminished healing capacity. It's also possible that untreated autoimmune conditions that persist for years may result in damage that eventually becomes permanent. Whatever the reason, this suggests that inflammation typically lingers much longer than would be expected (based on the absence of clinical symptoms), under the prevailing circumstances. And the result of course is much slower healing than most people (including many physicians) expect.

This phenomenon whereby the healing process becomes stuck in the first stage, is not limited to the inflammatory bowel diseases. It is apparently true for all autoimmune-associated diseases. The inflammation continues indefinitely because the healing process is prevented from proceeding normally. Some healing occurs, but it is repeatedly disrupted by new inflammation.

Summary

The main point to note in this chapter is that healing begins with inflammation and before it can proceed, existing dead or damaged cells and any other debris at the site must be removed by the specialized cells in the immune system that serve as the cleanup crew. If that step cannot be completed, then the process becomes stalled at this stage, and the progress of the healing cycle is effectively placed in a condition of indefinite hold as it waits for the cleanup process to be completed.

Chapter 3

Vitamin D Deficiency Has Been Shown to Be Linked With Many Autoimmune Diseases

Over 160 diseases have been classified as autoimmune, and the number continues to increase.

Hashimoto's thyroiditis was the first disease to be classified as autoimmune, and this determination was made in the year 1912. It's also known to be the most common cause of thyroid disease on the continent of North America. Recent research has shown that when compared with normal individuals, blood levels of vitamin D in the form of 25(OH)D (sometimes written as 25 hydroxy D), are typically much lower in people who have

Hashimoto's thyroiditis.[1] Not only that, but the longer they have had the disease, and the higher their antibody levels, the lower their blood levels of vitamin D tend to be. This suggests that a vitamin D deficiency may predispose to Hashimoto's thyroiditis, and conversely, Hashimoto's disease appears to contribute to a depletion of vitamin D levels in the body.

Diabetes mellitus is an increasing health problem in many countries.

Type 1 diabetes, typically diagnosed during childhood, is clearly an autoimmune disease. And the evidence indicates that type 2 diabetes is also autoimmune-associated.[2, 3] According to the results of a recent poll, approximately 1 in 8 American adults have been diagnosed with type 2 diabetes.[4] Based on the trend indicated by that poll, when compared with other data, type 2 diabetes appears to be one of the fastest growing diseases in America today. As is the case with many autoimmune diseases, victims often don't realize they're in trouble until clinical symptoms of the disease become obvious.

In a study of a group of United States active-duty military personnel, it was found that young, healthy, non-Hispanic white adults who had a vitamin D blood level of 40 ng/ml (100 nmol/l) or higher, were 44 % less likely to develop Type 1 diabetes, than their cohorts who had a vitamin D blood level of 30 ng/ml (75 nmol/l) or less.[5]

Note that 30 ng/ml (75 nmol/l) is the level that is officially recognized by most medical authorities to be the lower limit of the so-called "normal" range for vitamin D associated with optimal health. Obviously the results of this study bring into question the validity of the official guidelines followed by most medical professionals.

Even more puzzling is the fact that despite numerous research studies that have provided evidence such as the example described above, the prestigious Institute of Medicine insists that a vitamin D level of 20 ng/ml (50 nmol/l) is adequate for optimum health. And they even go on to claim that a 25(OH)D level greater than 50 ng/ml (125 nmol/l) could potentially have adverse effects.

Almost unbelievably, in the face of increasing research evidence to the contrary, the Institute of Medicine recently lowered their guideline for the minimum recommended level of vitamin D for optimum health to 20 ng/ml (50 nmol/l), from their earlier standard of 30 ng/ml (75 nmol/l). That change clearly conflicts with the findings of many current health studies.

While overdosing of any vitamin supplement should certainly not be taken lightly, in view of the latest research results confirmed by numerous studies, one has to wonder if some of the adverse effects from higher 25(OH)D levels that the Institute of Medicine warns about might be in reference to negative effects on hospital and physician income that could result from healthier consumers who no longer need as much remedial health care. After all, it seems rather obvious that 20 ng/ml (50 nmol/l) is clearly not an optimum vitamin D level. And it also appears that higher vitamin D levels are far more likely to help prevent disease, than to cause health problems. Diabetes is an increasing health problem in this country and in many other developed countries, so one has to wonder why the Institute of Medicine would adopt a recommendation that is clearly associated with an increased risk of developing diabetes, compared with recommending a higher level of vitamin D.

One of the oldest autoimmune diseases is rheumatoid arthritis.

The well-known Nurses Health Study, which began several decades ago, showed that women who lived in locations with higher ultraviolet B levels were significantly less likely to develop rheumatoid arthritis than women who lived in areas with lower average ultraviolet B levels. But a later study showed that after about the year 1980, that advantage no longer existed. Researchers concluded that the change was probably due to increasing use of sunscreen, resulting in less vitamin D being produced as a result of sun exposure.[6] In addition to showing that less sun exposure resulted in a higher risk of developing rheumatoid arthritis, these studies also showed that with less sun exposure, the disease began to develop at a much younger age, on the average.

Another study compared serum vitamin D levels of 54 rheumatoid arthritis patients in southern Europe (Italy) and 64 rheumatoid arthritis patients in northern Europe (Estonia) with serum vitamin D levels of normal healthy controls in each respective country.[7] The results showed that serum levels of vitamin D varied significantly with the seasons for all groups, but were consistently significantly higher in both winter and summer in Italian residents, compared with Estonian residents. Estonian patients had significantly lower average serum vitamin D levels, compared with Italian patients, and their vitamin D level varied with the seasons. Clinical symptoms for RA were more severe as vitamin D blood levels decreased, and this was true for patients in both northern and southern areas of Europe.

One of the more interesting findings of the study was that during the summer, increasing blood levels of vitamin D strongly correlated with decreasing disease activity levels of RA in Italian patients (but not in Estonian patients). And during the winter, decreasing blood levels of vitamin D strongly correlated with increasing disease activity levels of RA in Estonian patients (but not in Italian patients).

The authors of the study concluded that in general, blood levels of vitamin D were significantly lower in RA patients from North Europe when compared with RA patients from South Europe, and they varied with summer and winter, for both locations. This suggests that in Estonia (with less effective sunlight exposure in the summer, due to the higher latitude, vitamin D levels did not rise to a high enough level during summer to strongly suppress RA symptoms.

But the most important finding for our purposes in this book, was that blood levels of vitamin D show a significant inverse correlation with RA disease activity levels in RA patients from both North and South Europe. Simply put, the higher the blood level of vitamin D, the lower the severity of RA symptoms. And conversely, the lower the blood level of vitamin D, the more severe the RA symptoms.

Multiple sclerosis is another debilitating disease with autoimmune origins.

One of the first neurological markers of multiple sclerosis (MS) to appear for many patients is known (in medical terms) as a "clinically isolated syndrome" (CIS). A common example of a CIS is optic neuritis (inflammation of the optic nerve, often resulting in pain, numbness, or tingling). When a CIS is detected, an MRI of the brain is usually ordered to rule out lesions. If they are detected, the presence of lesions indicates a very high risk of developing MS. Roughly half of all patients who have optic neuritis, eventually develop MS. Obviously, at this stage any effective preventative measures can be extremely valuable.

When lesions are present, associated with a CIS, the cause of inflammation is typically due to an attack by the immune system on the myelin sheaths that protect and insulate nerve fibers. This is known as a "demyelinating" event, and it is the reason why MS is classified as a demyelinating disease. In fact, MS is the most common demyelinating disease. Typically, when a second demyelinating event occurs, a diagnosis of MS is established.

With demyelinating diseases, if sufficient damage accrues over time to the myelin sheaths, the nerves that they originally protected, will die. When that happens, the damage cannot be reversed.

But research exists to demonstrate that the progression of CIS events to MS can be delayed and possibly postponed indefinitely in some cases. In a double-blind, randomized trial in which the subjects had all been diagnosed with optic neuritis, and who had a 25(OH)D blood level below 30 ng/ml (75 nmol/l), Derakhshandi et al. (2013) were able to show that vitamin D is very effective at reducing the risk level.[8] The vitamin D group received 50,000 IU of vitamin D per week (which is equivalent to roughly 7,000 IU per day), while the other group received a placebo.

Of the group that received the vitamin D supplement, not a single person experienced a second demyelinating event. On the other hand, almost half of the group that received a placebo experienced a demyelinating event (5 out of 11), and therefore they progressed to a diagnosis of MS. The researchers concluded that the protection provided by the vitamin D supplement in this particular study led to a 68.4 % risk reduction, overall. Compared with most preventive medical treatments in general, that is a very high rate of success.

Recent research shows that autistic children produce antibodies against their own brain tissue, and the condition appears to be associated with vitamin D deficiency.

In fact, 70 % of the autistic subjects in a study were producing anti-myelin-associated glycoprotein (anti-MAG) auto-antibodies.[9] And while the subjects in the control group ("normal" children) had an average vitamin D level of 33 ng/ml (82 nmol/l), the

35

autistic group averaged only 14 ng/ml (35 nmol/l), well down in the deficiency range. So it appears that in addition to possibly being another demyelinating disease, autism may be a disease of vitamin D deficiency. This is emphasized by the authors' observation that, "The results of this study may indicate that 25-hydroxy vitamin D deficiency may be a possible contributing factor to the increased frequency of serum anti-MAG auto-antibodies in some autistic children" (Mostafa and AL-Ayadhi, 2012. p. 201).

But this is not the first study to suggest that autism might be the result of an autoimmune condition, so it shouldn't be surprising that vitamin D deficiency might be associated with the production of antibodies that target brain tissue in autistic children. An earlier study showed that over 70 % of autistic children were deficient in regulatory T-cells.[10] That's an important finding, since regulatory T-cells normally play a critical role in preventing the development of autoimmune syndromes (by helping to maintain a state of immunological self-tolerance).

Inflammatory bowel disease is also known to be associated with vitamin D deficiency.

Research shows that the development of inflammatory bowel disease is commonly associated with vitamin D deficiency.[11] And additionally, inflammatory bowel disease tends to deplete vitamin D levels in the body, thereby compounding the problem.[12]

Many additional autoimmune diseases have been associated with vitamin D deficiency.

Some examples include osteoarthritis, Addison's disease, autoimmune hepatitis, asthma, periodontitis, psoriasis, and amyotrophic lateral sclerosis (ALS). This is only a partial list, and the list will surely continue to grow as more research is done.

Summary

As the examples discussed in this chapter illustrate, vitamin D deficiency has already been shown to be associated with many well-known autoimmune-associated syndromes, and current research continues to provide additional evidence of a similar association with additional autoimmune diseases.

Chapter 4

Many Non-Autoimmune Diseases Are Also Associated With Vitamin D Deficiency

Cancer is a well-known example of a non-autoimmune disease that has been shown to be associated with vitamin D deficiency.

Though the survival rates of cancer patients for many of the various types of cancer appear to be slowly but steadily improving, that doesn't mean that cancer is becoming less of a threat. While the diagnostic rate of some types seems to be declining, by contrast, other types of cancer are clearly on the increase, according to the latest published data from the National Cancer Institute's

Vitamin D Deficiency and Autoimmune Disease

Center to Reduce Cancer Health Disparities.[1] In fact, many types of cancer are more common today than ever before in history.

Worldwide, one of the most common forms of upper gastrointestinal malignancies is esophageal cancer. A study was recently done in China to evaluate the roles of vitamin D and beta-carotene (BC) in the development of esophageal squamous cell cancer.[2] Vitamin D and beta-carotene blood levels were compared for 100 newly-diagnosed esophageal cancer patients and 200 healthy controls, matched by age, sex, and area of residence. It was found that the blood levels of both vitamin D and beta-carotene were significantly lower in the newly-diagnosed patients, when compared with the controls. The researchers concluded that:

> *In conclusions [sic], our finding provides important evidences [sic] that a reduced risk of esophageal cancer may be associated with increased circulating concentrations of VD3 and BC. But it is not significantly associated with the dietary BC intake. This study suggests that BC and VD3 are the protective factors for esophageal cancer.*(Huang et al., 2014, p. 823)

Since beta-carotene intake had no significant effect, that suggests that either developing cancer or vitamin D deficiency may suppress blood levels of beta-carotene. It also implies that a low serum vitamin D level may have a more significant effect than a low serum beta-carotene level.

40

In a recent study that involved following more than 4,000 breast cancer patients over an average period of 9 years, researchers determined that high blood levels of vitamin D cut the mortality risk in half, compared with low blood levels of vitamin D.[3] The results were so compelling that the researchers recommended that doctors treating cancer patients should consider adding supplemental vitamin D to their patients' treatment programs immediately, rather than to follow the usual practice of waiting for additional research to confirm the findings, before making recommendations to modify existing treatment programs.

Vitamin D deficiency has been shown to be associated with a broad range of pediatric health issues.

Blood levels of vitamin D don't have to be low enough to be in the deficiency range (below 20 ng/ml [50 nmol/l]) to cause problems. Researchers have found that kids who have vitamin D blood levels below the sufficiency level (30 ng/ml [50 nmol/l]) have almost twice the risk of being anemic, compared with kids who have adequate vitamin D levels.[4]

The cause of defects in the enamel of the teeth of very young children (defects that lead to the development of cavities) has been traced to their mothers' vitamin D levels, while they were still in the womb.[5]

In a study of mentally ill adolescents, Gracious, Finucane, Friedman-Campbell, Messing, and Parkhurst (2012) showed that an astonishing 72 % of adolescents with psychotic issues, had either deficient or insufficient vitamin D blood levels.[6]

Research data suggest that Alzheimer's disease may be caused by a vitamin D deficiency.

In fact, research shows that 70–90 % of Alzheimer's patients are deficient in vitamin D.[7] Surely such a high correlation has to be much more than a mere coincidence. Though they don't understand exactly how it does so, some researchers are convinced that vitamin D protects the brain from Alzheimer's disease.[8] Furthermore, it appears that the medications typically used to treat Alzheimer's disease tend to increase the body's ability to absorb vitamin D. This suggests that enhanced vitamin D absorption might possibly be the main reason why the medications are effective in treating the disease.[9]

You probably recall that back in chapter 3 (pages 31–33) we discussed how vitamin D is effective at preventing the development of multiple sclerosis. Apparently it prevents MS by preventing demyelinating issues from progressing, as demonstrated by research done by Derakhshandi et al. (2013).[10] The relatively high correlation of vitamin D deficiency with Alzheimer's disease suggests that Alzheimer's may possibly also be a demyelinating disease. In fact, researchers (Carmeli et al., 2013) have discovered that demyelination can be found in the very earliest stages of dementia, when only mild cognitive impairment is present. This suggests that the presence of this type of damage to the nerve sheaths may set the stage for the development of Alzheimer's disease as the demyelination process progresses.[11]

Non-Alzheimer's dementia is also associated with vitamin D deficiency.

In France, a 7-year research study showed that women who were significantly vitamin D deficient (average hydroxyvitamin D level less than 10 ng/ml) (25 nmol/l) at the start of the study were almost 20 times more likely to develop non-Alzheimer's dementia than women whose hydroxyvitamin D level was above 10 ng/ml (25 nmol/l).[12]

And results were recently published for a very interesting study in which scientists were attempting to determine whether vitamin D deficiency is associated with both Alzheimer's disease and dementia that can be attributed to all other causes.[13]

After selecting 1,658 elderly subjects who initially had no history of dementia, cardiovascular disease, or stroke, and measuring their initial serum vitamin D levels, Littlejohns et. al. (2014) analyzed dementia and Alzheimer's status of the subjects approximately 6 years later (actual mean follow-up interval was 5.6 years). They found 102 cases of Alzheimer's disease and 171 cases of dementia attributable to other causes. The researchers determined that a serum vitamin D level below 20 mg/dl dramatically increased the risk of developing either Alzheimer's disease or all-cause dementia.

Vitamin D is essential for maintaining bone density.

By now the importance of an adequate vitamin D blood level regarding the prevention of osteoporosis is relatively well known.[14] Good bone density can only be maintained if an adequate supply of vitamin D and an adequate amount of magnesium is available in the diet, because without these essential elements, calcium cannot be properly absorbed and utilized, regardless of how much calcium might be in the diet, or how much might be taken as a supplement. Most diets (in developed countries) contain more than enough calcium for strong and healthy bones, provided that adequate amounts of vitamin D and magnesium are maintained.

It's interesting to note that the developed countries that have the highest levels of calcium intake also have the highest rates of osteoporosis. It seems likely that the fact that those countries also appear to be experiencing an epidemic of vitamin D deficiency is probably more than just a coincidence.

Older adults who are at risk of falling can be helped by vitamin D.

Research conducted in France has demonstrated that higher levels of vitamin D (levels well above the arbitrarily-designated "sufficient" level) can improve balance in older adults, thereby reducing the risk of falls in this age group.[15] In this particular study, those who had the highest vitamin D levels (around 55 ng/ml [137 nmol/l]) had significantly better balance when compared with those who had barely sufficient levels in the 30–55 ng/ml (75–137 nmol/l) range. It's unfortunate that subjects who had even higher vitamin D levels were not available for testing, because this leaves us wondering if higher levels might be associated with even better balance characteristics.

Vitamin D affects many organs in the body.

In order for vitamin D to have an effect, vitamin D receptors must be present of course. Vitamin D receptors (VDRs) can be found in bone, skeletal muscle, heart muscle, cartilage, intestines, brain, thyroid, adrenals, kidneys, liver, reproductive organs, retina, hair follicles, fat tissue, and other organs. In addition, researchers have pinpointed at least 2,776 locations in the human genome where vitamin D receptors can be found, and they have determined that vitamin D receptors can change the expression of at least 229 genes, in response to vitamin D.[16] That's an extremely broad range of influence, to say the least. The ability to alter gene expression carries almost incomprehensible significance.

Vitamin D deficiency has often been mis-diagnosed.

At least one researcher (Holick, 2004), who has described in detail the importance of how vitamin D prevents the development of cancers, type 1 diabetes, heart disease, and osteoporosis, has pointed out that, "Vitamin D deficiency is often misdiagnosed as fibromyalgia" (p. 362).[17] And a sad reflection on the inexcusable lack of familiarity of many doctors today with the old disease of rickets, is the fact that many cases of childhood rickets (which is caused by vitamin D deficiency) are misdiagnosed as child abuse.[18] That smacks of incompetence of the worst kind, since it typically results in innocent parents being prosecuted for child abuse that never happened, while the children are traumatized by being taken away from their parents and placed under the care of State protective child custody services.

Above all, vitamin D is important for longevity.

There's no question that the best source of vitamin D is the sun, and utilizing the sun to produce vitamin D on the surface of the skin is generally preferred over supplementation, whenever sun exposure is an option. And when it comes to living longer and living healthier, nothing provides more bang for our buck than vitamin D. Researchers who recently published data describing a 20-year follow-up study of almost 30,000 Swedish women, discovered that the women in the study who avoided sun exposure typically experienced almost double the overall mortality rate of women who received the highest rates of sun exposure.[19] They concluded that:

> *The results of this study provide observational evidence that avoiding sun exposure is a risk factor for all-cause mortality. Following sun exposure advice that is very restrictive in countries with low solar intensity might in fact be harmful to women's health.* (Lindqvist et al., 2014, p. 77)

Many other health issues are also associated with inadequate vitamin D levels.

These include (but are not necessarily limited to) osteoporosis, osteopenia, spinal ossification, and other causes of loss of bone density, various cardiovascular issues, immune system diseases, metabolic diseases, cirrhosis of the liver, susceptibility to infections such as AIDS, Q fever, leprosy, and tuberculosis, kidney disease, neurological disorders, and growth disorders such as low birth weight and low body mass.

We can micro-analyze our nutritional and vitamin intake until our head spins, but the bottom line is that we live longer (and healthier) if we make sure that our vitamin D level is up where it needs to be. If we don't take the time to do that, we may actually be shortening our lifespan without even realizing it.

Summary
The list of health issues that can be minimized or eliminated by a sufficiently-high serum vitamin D level is quite long, and growing almost daily. From horrific diseases such as cancer, to widely-varying issues such as osteoporosis, mental health, anemia, and balance problems, vitamin D is important for the health and well-being of virtually every organ in the body.

The fact that vitamin D can even alter the expression of at least 229 genes means that it plays a vital role in many aspects of our health. And the icing on the cake is the probability that by keeping our vitamin D level up in the safe range, we will very likely live longer and we will live healthier, which implies that we will live happier.

Chapter 5

Exactly How Does Vitamin D Deficiency Lead to Autoimmune Disease?

The role of vitamin D in apoptosis.

On a microscopic basis, human tissue is composed of individual cells. The cells in most organs in the body are replaced by new cells on a regular schedule. Whenever the existing cells exceed a certain age, or if they have somehow become damaged, or diseased, or their ability to function normally is otherwise impaired, they are replaced by new cells. The replacement schedule varies widely, typically depending on the environment to which the organ is exposed, and the duties that it performs. Except for the hippocampus portion, the brain seems to be an exception to this rule, and most authorities believe that (with the exception noted) the brain cells that we are born with, remain with us for our entire lifetime.

Vitamin D Deficiency and Autoimmune Disease

For example, the cells in the mucosal lining of the stomach are normally replaced on a schedule of approximately every 2 days. This is necessary because of the harsh, extremely acidic environment to which the cells are exposed when digesting food. Cells in the lining of the small intestine are subjected to duties that are not quite as hazardous as the digestive processes that occur in the stomach. For one thing, most of the acidity of the chyme (partially-digested food that has passed into the small intestine from the stomach) has been mostly neutralized by the addition of bicarbonate released from the pancreas. And so the cells in the lining of the small intestine are normally replaced about every 4 to 6 days. The cells in most other organs are typically replaced less often. As an example, the cells in the skin (the epidermis) are replaced about once each month.

When the immune system recognizes that a cell needs to be replaced, it marks that cell for destruction. After the cell is destroyed, and the residue is disposed of, the growth of a new replacement cell can occur. Replacement cells are generated by means of cell division, but since the details of that process are not particularly relevant to our discussion, we won't explore those details here. If a brief review of the process is desired, there are many sources available for this type of information.[1, 2]

The mechanism by which cells are marked for destruction (and subsequently destroyed) is known as apoptosis, and it's a vital part of the healing process for human tissue. Apoptosis is essentially programmed cell death. It's the beginning step in the organ repair and maintenance routine, and it's carried out under the supervision of the immune system.

But as noted in chapter 2, when autoimmune disease is present, the self-perpetuating nature of the reaction cycle tends to prevent the healing process from getting past the inflammation stage, and healing cannot proceed normally. The important question of course is, "Exactly why is the healing process prevented from proceeding as nature intended?" And the answer to that question appears to involve vitamin D — specifically, inadequate availability of vitamin D.

Could it be that simple?
The research data suggest that it certainly might be. Researchers investigating the relationship between blood levels of vitamin D and systemic lupus erythematosus (SLE), have uncovered some very compelling evidence. They discovered that out of a group of 290 SLE patients, 96 % of them had a blood level of vitamin D [25(OH)D(3)] that would qualify as insufficiency (below 30 ng/ml [75 nmol/l]).[3] 27 % of them had a vitamin D blood level that would qualify as a serious deficiency (below 15 ng/ml [37 nmol/l]). 96 % is an extremely high correlation rate for any type of scientific study, so this is a very impressive level of correlation.

Does this prove that low vitamin D is the cause of SLE?
No, of course not. While it provides a very strong association, it does not constitute scientific proof. But it does point to an apparent "smoking gun", and it certainly provides us with some inspiring insight to suggest that it might be prudent for us to keep

Vitamin D Deficiency and Autoimmune Disease

our blood levels of vitamin D well above 30 ng/ml (75 nmol/l), lest we find ourselves unwittingly becoming one more case in the SLE statistics (in the event that our genes happen to make us vulnerable to the development of SLE). Obviously this does not imply that everyone who has a low vitamin D blood level will develop SLE. That can only happen if certain other conditions are met, beginning with certain predisposing genetic requirements.

But just because this research was specifically directed at an association between vitamin D and SLE does not by any means imply that similar associations do not exist between blood levels of vitamin D and other autoimmune diseases (nor does it imply that such associations do exist). Clearly, I am not alone in believing that vitamin D may play a key role in the development of not just SLE, but possibly all autoimmune type diseases. In an editorial also published in Rheumatology, other researchers, Munoz et al. (2011), have speculated that:[4]

> *Considering these robust epidemiological data, one might believe that vitamin D deficiency plays a pivotal role in the multifaceted aetiopathogenesis of autoimmunity that deserves further scientific research to pinpoint the mechanisms of action of vitamin D in the phagocytosis and clearance of dying cells. (p. 586)*

"Aetiopathogenesis" is a medical term that refers to the origination of, and the development of, an abnormal condition or disease. Phagocytes are a certain type of white blood cell, such as neutrophils or macrophages, that are uniquely designed to do a special job, namely to capture, ingest, or engulf other cells, pathogens, particles, or debris, in order to destroy the items and remove them from the body. The process of doing this is known as phagocytosis. According to the editorial mentioned above (Munoz et al., 2011), the authors' position is based on the observation that with SLE at least, the presence of an adequate level of properly-executed phagocytosis is necessary for the removal of cells marked for apoptosis.

In order to establish a better understanding of the process of phagocytosis, a short but very fascinating video of a neutrophil chasing and capturing a bacterium (Staphylococcus aureus) around and among red blood cells in blood can be viewed at the following URL. This video was created from a 16-mm movie, originally made in the 1950s. It was filmed through a microscope, at Vanderbilt University, by the late David Rogers, and it does an excellent job of portraying the process of phagocytosis.[5]

http://sciencehack.com/videos/view/I_xh-bkiv_c

Researchers believe that SLE can be triggered when the healing process becomes stalled.

It is believed that when those apoptotic cells cannot be removed, SLE can be triggered, or if it has already been triggered, symptoms are likely to become worse (Munoz et al., 2011). In other words, as the debris accumulates, the inflammation associated with the disease is either sustained, or exacerbated. This has been verified by numerous experiments (references are cited by the research article).

It has been previously demonstrated that in normal, healthy subjects, vitamin D greatly enhances the ability of phagocytes to perform.[6] The key point of interest here then is the observation that without adequate vitamin D, phagocytosis cannot proceed normally, and therefore inflammatory debris tends to accumulate so that the cycle of events and the chronic inflammation eventually lead to a self-perpetuating, autoimmune type reaction. Thus it seems quite possible that an inadequate blood level of vitamin D might lead to the development of autoimmune disease. But obviously this is still epidemiological evidence (albeit strong evidence), and does not constitute scientific proof.

2 alternative forms of vitamin D supplements exist.

Note that the research articles cited here refer to vitamin D3, rather than just plain vitamin D. In fact, 2 forms of vitamin D are commonly available — vitamin D2 and vitamin D3. Vitamin D2 is otherwise known as ergocalciferol, and vitamin D3 is known as cholecalciferol. Interestingly, when physicians prescribe vitamin D, the prescriptions almost invariably refer to vitamin D2, but by contrast, virtually all of the over-the-counter vitamin D supplements are in the form of vitamin D3.

Many decades ago, vitamin D2 was thought to be the equivalent of vitamin D3, but that assumption can no longer be justified. Why physicians continue to prescribe vitamin D2 is somewhat of a mystery, since research shows that vitamin D3 supplements are consistently more effective than vitamin D2 supplements. Houghton and Vieth, (2006), summed up the case against vitamin D2 supplements with this statement:[7]

> The case that vitamin D2 should no longer be considered equivalent to vitamin D3 is based on differences in their efficacy at raising serum 25-hydroxyvitamin D, diminished binding of vitamin D2 metabolites to vitamin D binding protein in plasma, and a nonphysiologic metabolism and shorter shelf life of vitamin D2. Vitamin D2, or ergocalciferol, should not be regarded as a nutrient suitable for supplementation or fortification. (p. 696)

Therefore for our purposes in this book, please be aware that we will ignore vitamin D2 for all practical purposes. For convenience, we will use the terms "vitamin D" and "vitamin D3" interchangeably, as if they are one and the same. In other words, anytime you see the term "vitamin D" in this book, assume that it implies "vitamin D3".

Additional validation of the evidence that vitamin D deficiency is a key risk factor for autoimmunity can be found in other research concerning antinuclear antibodies. It is known that individuals who test positive for antinuclear antibodies (ANA-positive) are at a significant risk of developing SLE.

A compelling case for the effectiveness of vitamin D in preventing the development of autoimmunity can be found in the discovery that even ANA-positive healthy controls are more likely to have lower blood levels of vitamin D than ANA-negative healthy controls.[8] In other words, those individuals who have pre-condition markers that qualify them as candidates for the development of SLE (but who do not yet have the disease) typically have a lower blood level of vitamin D than those who do not have the markers that indicate that they are predisposed to the development of SLE.

Vitamin D becomes biologically active by binding to vitamin D receptors.

As mentioned on page 40 in chapter 3, not much can happen until vitamin D transfers it's health benefits to the body by binding to vitamin D receptors (VDRs). VDRs can be found at various locations in the body, in the cells of the tissues of most organs, including bone, brain, breast, gonads, heart, intestines, kidneys, prostate, parathyroids, and skin, for example.

Vitamin D receptor numbers tend to be concentrated around genes associated with cancer and autoimmunity.

To further illuminate how vitamin D (or vitamin D deficiency) influences cancer and autoimmune disease development, Ramagopalan et al. (2010), as part of a genome-wide map of vitamin D receptor binding, found that:[9]

> *VDR binding sites were significantly enriched near autoimmune and cancer associated genes identified from genome-wide association (GWA) studies. Notable genes with VDR binding*

> *included IRF8, associated with MS, and PTPN2 associated with Crohn's disease and T1D. Furthermore, a number of single nucleotide polymorphism associations from GWA were located directly within VDR binding intervals, for example, rs13385731 associated with SLE and rs947474 associated with T1D.* (p. 1352)

In that quote, MS stands for multiple sclerosis, T1D stands for type 1 diabetes, and SLE stands for systemic lupus erythematosus. In other words, the researchers found that vitamin D receptors were present in much greater numbers in the vicinity of genes associated with cancer and autoimmune diseases. This clearly indicates that vitamin D plays an important role in the expression of these genes. We have already discussed the autoimmune origins of multiple sclerosis, Crohn's disease, type 1 diabetes, and systemic lupus erythematosus in chapter 3. Note that genes associated with the development of these particular diseases are specifically mentioned in the quote above, as being sites of increased numbers of vitamin D receptors.

Vitamin D is initially in an inactive form.

Vitamin D, whether produced by the action of sunlight on skin, ingested in food, or absorbed from a vitamin D supplement, is initially in an inactive form. After it is processed by the liver, (by hydroxylation) it is commonly designated as 25(OH)D(3), or simply 25(OH)D. But this is still an inactive form. Before our body can utilize it, vitamin D has to be converted into the active form, $1,25(OH)_2D3$. This process is normally completed in the kidneys, after it is initiated in the liver.

Vitamin D Deficiency and Autoimmune Disease

Technically, as we shall see later in this chapter (on page 55), a small percentage of 25(OH)D is converted into 1,25(OH)$_2$D by mast cells. But the lion's share is converted in the kidneys. The active form of vitamin D is extremely potent, but very short--lived.

For a detailed description, here's how the National Institutes of Health Office of Dietary Supplements describes the conversion of vitamin D from the inactive form to the active form that can be utilized by the body:[10]

> *Vitamin D is a fat-soluble vitamin that is naturally present in very few foods, added to others, and available as a dietary supplement. It is also produced endogenously when ultraviolet rays from sunlight strike the skin and trigger vitamin D synthesis. Vitamin D obtained from sun exposure, food, and supplements is biologically inert and must undergo two hydroxylations in the body for activation. The first occurs in the liver and converts vitamin D to 25-hydroxyvitamin D [25(OH)D], also known as calcidiol. The second occurs primarily in the kidney and forms the physiologically active 1,25-dihydroxyvitamin D [1,25(OH)$_2$D], also known as calcitriol [1].*

Note that the active form is sometimes written as 1α,25(OH)2D3, or 1α,25(OH)$_2$D3. Perhaps this is a good place to mention that when ordering a vitamin D test for a patient, doctors sometimes mistakenly order a test for the active form, 1,25(OH)$_2$D3, instead of the correct test, for 25(OH)D. Ordering the wrong type of test can lead to much confusion about the patient's actual vitamin D status, because a high result on the 1,25(OH)$_2$D3 test can occur in conjunction with active autoimmune disease when in fact the 25(OH)D level is actually quite low.

This condition apparently develops due to the likelihood that the body will continue to convert large amounts of vitamin D into the active form, in order to meet the needs of the immune system as the immune system attempts to control chronic inflammation and/or disease. This places abnormally high demands on the available supply, and as a result the 25(OH)D level can run low if a higher than normal amount of vitamin D is not regularly resupplied by sun exposure, diet, or supplementation. Therefore when requesting a vitamin D test, always make sure that your doctor orders the 25(OH)D test. This is pronounced, "twenty-five hydroxy D", or "twenty-five hydroxyvitamin D".

The active form of vitamin D is much more potent than the inactive form.

While we are discussing these 2 forms of vitamin D, it should be noted that the VDRs are capable of binding to several forms of vitamin D3. However, their affinity for $1,25(OH)_2D3$ (the active form) is roughly 1,000 times as great as it is for 25(OH)D (an inactive form). And in a nutshell, this defines why the active form of vitamin D3 is so much more potent than the inactive form.

As we have already discussed, chronic inflammation leads to the development of autoimmune disease. So how does this relate to the association between inflammation and vitamin D? Well, we know that human mast cells are not only loaded with proinflammatory agents, but we also know from research published by Yip et al. (2014) that mast cells are capable of converting 25(OH)D into the active form, $1,25(OH)_2D3$.[11]

Furthermore, we know that research results published by Yip et al. (2014) show that both the inactive and the active forms of vitamin D3 are capable of suppressing mast cell degranulation (that would otherwise result in the release of proinflammatory mediators) caused by classic allergic reactions. And we know that this response (the suppression of mast cell degranulation) depends on the activation of vitamin D receptors.

Now the situation is getting interesting.

As we review more recently-published research data, we can begin to see all sorts of connections to confirm what we have been suspecting. Way back in chapter 1 we discussed how mast cells release proinflammatory modulators when they are activated. And as we noted above, mast cells are capable of converting vitamin D3 into the active form, $1,25(OH)_2D3$. Researchers in Italy (Baroni et al., 2007) have shown that $1,25(OH)_2D3$ also plays a role in the regulation of the development and function of mast cells.[12]

So mast cells regulate vitamin D, and vitamin D regulates mast cells.

Specifically, mast cells can regulate the conversion of vitamin D from the inactive to the active form, and the active form of of vitamin D can regulate mast cells, by limiting their development. Baroni et al. (2007) showed that the active form of vitamin D not only initiates apoptosis, but it is also capable of limiting (in a dose-dependent manner) the ability of mast cell precursors to mature (into fully-capable mast cells), dependent upon the presence of vitamin D receptors.

It doesn't get much more co-dependent, convoluted, and generally complex than that. Furthermore, Baroni et al. (2007) also demonstrated that VDR-deficient mice experience faster mast cell maturity rates than normal mice, and the mast cells that are produced are more easily-activated, compared with those produced by normal mice.

Is it any wonder then that so many people, including many professionals, are confused about how the immune system actually works?

It's a very complex and sophisticated system. And it can do wonderful things for us, provided that we just do our part to help keep it functioning properly. What this interdependent relationship implies then, is that vitamin D receptors must be present in adequate quantities in order for the active form of vitamin D to be able to prevent the production of excess numbers of mast cells when an inflammatory event is in progress. This is a mechanism that the immune system utilizes to prevent reactions from getting out of hand.

This is so important that I'm going to emphasize it by repeating it. There must be a sufficient number of vitamin D receptors present, and a sufficient amount of the active form of vitamin D must be available, so that the production and inappropriate activation of mast cells will be prevented from reaching a level at which excessive inflammation is generated, far above the amount normally associated with such an event.

This phenomenon appears to explain why so many IBD patients tend to have mast cell activation disorder.

Mast cell activation disorder (MCAD) is a condition marked by inappropriate mast cell activation that results in the excessive release of histamine, cytokines, and other proinflammatory mediators by mast cells, for no legitimate (or at least no apparent) reason. It can cause many of the symptoms of mastocytosis or mastocytic enterocolitis, even though mast cell populations might be normal, or only slightly elevated.

While mastocytic enterocolitis is a form of microscopic colitis marked by excessive mast cell numbers in the intestines, mastocytosis is a systemic disease marked by a chronic state of excessive mast cell numbers in multiple organs, or even all organs, in the body. It causes episodes of excessive inflammation that can be initiated by various seemingly-unrelated triggers such as heat, sunlight, exercise, chemical odors, or other causes.

MCAD, by contrast, is not normally associated with a chronic condition of excessive numbers of mast cells. While mast cell counts may be elevated at times, in some cases, many cases of MCAD involve only normal numbers of mast cells, but for some unknown reason, many of the mast cells degranulate for no ob-

vious reason. By doing so, they create an inflammatory state
that should not exist.

The intestines are known to have relatively high populations of
mast cells, thus they are fertile sites for mast cell-induced inflammation. MCAD can result in additional symptoms of the type
normally associated with IgE-based reactions that cause compli-
cations and add confounding issues to certain types of autoimmune diseases, such as inflammatory bowel disease. IgE-based
reactions are relatively short-lived reactions that result when IgE
antibodies are produced by the immune system, which prompts
mast cells to release histamine into the bloodstream. The histamine leads to the familiar symptoms that most of us are familiar with that are triggered by pollen, dust, and mold, for example

In the case of microscopic colitis (of which lymphocytic colitis
and collagenous colitis are the most common types) for example,
MCAD appears to be capable of causing virtually any of the clinical gastroenterological symptoms traditionally associated with
the disease, plus the addition of classic IgE-based allergy symptoms such as nasal discharge, watery eyes, and itching skin or
tongue, in some cases. These symptoms are usually somewhat
attenuated (compared with classic allergic reactions), and they
may even be overlooked, unless the patient is aware of this possibility, and remains alert, in order to notice the symptoms.

But whether these symptoms are relatively minor, or severe, the
additional mast cell activity typically results in increased severi-

Vitamin D Deficiency and Autoimmune Disease

ty of gastrointestinal symptoms normally associated with an IBD, and in some situations, this type of mast cell activity can even trigger a flare when an IBD has been in remission. And unlike classic allergies, which can be triggered by exposure to allergins in the airways, on the skin, or on the mucosal tissues of the mouth or esophagus, the IgE- based reactions that are sometimes associated with microscopic colitis are often triggered in the intestines.

The observations noted in the above paragraph are based on an ongoing epidemiological study of hundreds of people who have microscopic colitis and who share their experiences freely as members of an Internet discussion and support group.[13] This collection of real-life experiences is arguably the largest database in the world of specific information devoted to the understanding and treatment of microscopic colitis and related issues. The discussion board has been active (including continued participation by many of the original founding members) for approximately 10 years at this point in time, so a lot of real-life data are available.

Presumably, this effect may also apply to the other IBDs, including Crohn's, ulcerative colitis, and celiac disease, although this possibility certainly hasn't yet been verified by random, double-blind research trials. Not all IBD patients experience these IgE-based symptoms, but for those who do, this observation should answer a lot of questions.

So a deficiency of either vitamin D receptors, or vitamin D in it's active form can lead to a hypersensitive condition where not only are mast cells more likely to degranulate (releasing proin-flammatory agents), but additional mast cells are produced more rapidly, and more of them are ultimately produced, so that a state of severe hypersensitivity (resulting in massive inflammation) may be the result. This condition appears to meet the definition of at least mast cell activation disorder, and as already mentioned, it might possibly be the primary cause of mastocytic enterocolitis.

Other researchers have validated this discovery, and demonstrated how powerful the effect of vitamin D can be.

Additional compelling data about the association between vitamin D receptors and inflammation were established when Kong et al. (2008) showed that when normal mice, and mice with compromised vitamin D receptor function, were fed dextran sodium sulfate in order to intentionally attempt to induce colitis, the mice with compromised vitamin D receptors developed much more severe symptoms than the mice with normal vitamin D receptors.[14] The mortality rate in the mice with compromised VDR function ranged up to 70 %, whereas there was no mortality, and only relatively minor symptoms in the mice with normal VDR function. Needless to say, that's a striking difference in the results displayed by the comparison of the 2 groups of test subjects. And it indicates that the vitamin D receptors are capable of providing a powerful protective effect against inflammation in the intestines.

Vitamin D Deficiency and Autoimmune Disease

During a colonoscopy exam, gastroenterologists often take biopsy samples of the interior lining (known as the epithelia) of the colon, and these samples are later examined under a microscope by a pathologist in order to search for microscopic physical changes in the structure of the cells. Certain specific changes are considered to be diagnostic of certain digestive system diseases.

Researchers have shown that patients who have Crohn's disease and ulcerative colitis are indeed deficient in VDRs.

Liu et al. (2013) studied colonic biopsies in order to compare the status of vitamin D receptors in Crohn's disease and ulcerative colitis patients with the VDR status of normal subjects. Compared with the relatively high quantities of vitamin D receptors found in normal colonic epithelial tissue, the researchers found that Crohn's disease and ulcerative colitis were associated with a significant reduction in the number of VDRs.[15] By utilizing gene splicing techniques in mouse intestinal epithelial tissue, they demonstrated that a sufficient number of human VDRs expressed in mouse intestinal epithelial cells will protect mice from developing colitis.

The researchers concluded that, "Together, these results demonstrate that gut epithelial VDR signaling inhibits colitis by protecting the mucosal epithelial barrier, and this anticolitic activity is independent of nonepithelial immune VDR actions" (p. 3,982) (Liu et al. 2013). Obviously this is an extremely important observation, as it provides compelling evidence of a possible way to prevent the development of inflammatory bowel disease.

Exactly How Does Vitamin D Deficiency Lead to Autoimmune Disease?

In essence, the researchers have demonstrated that an adequate level of vitamin D (and sufficient numbers of vitamin D receptors) can prevent the development of inflammatory bowel disease. And if this is true in the gut, then there is good reason to believe that future research may verify that it is also true in other organs (including joints) affected by autoimmune-associated inflammation.

Vitamin D is actually a hormone.

In fact, the active form of vitamin D, $1,25(OH)_2D3$, is a steroid hormone, while the inactive form, $25(OH)D3$, can be described as a precursor to a hormone. But before hormones can serve any useful purpose in the body, they must be able to relay their molecular information and instructions, and they do this by binding to specialized proteins called receptors. In humans (and in fact in all vertebrates), there are five major categories of steroid hormone receptors. They are known as androgen receptors, estrogen receptors, glucocorticoid receptors, mineralocorticoid receptors, and progestin receptors.

Each type is specialized to match the needs of the hormones that it binds with. In the case of the glucocorticoid receptors, they contain nuclear receptors, and this is important to our discussion here, because the active form of vitamin D is a nuclear hormone. For anyone not familiar with this designation, no, a "nuclear" hormone is not radioactive. "Nuclear", in this case, simply refers to the fact that cells in this group are of a type that have a membrane-enclosed nucleus that contains most of their genetic material.

Vitamin D Deficiency and Autoimmune Disease

The unique characteristic of nuclear receptors that distinguishes them from other types of receptors is their ability to directly bind with DNA and to modify gene expression. For the purposes of this discussion, we only need to know a few basic facts about genes. First we need to recognize that a gene is a small segment of specially coded genetic material known as DNA. DNA stands for deoxyribonucleic acid, and almost every cell in the body contains identical DNA. Each gene contains a set of instructions for constructing molecules that are needed for reproduction and survival. And we need to know that gene expression is the process by which the information contained within a gene is utilized to produce a useful product.

Nuclear receptors are able to sense and bind to certain hormones such as cortisol, thyroid, and vitamin D. These hormones act as ligands and activate the respective receptors. For biological purposes, a ligand is simply a substance (typically a small molecule) that binds with a biologically-active (meaning that it is produced by a living organism) molecule in order to form a complex that serves a biological purpose.

Since nuclear receptors have the ability to bind directly to DNA, this means that when they are properly activated, the receptors are able to regulate the expression of adjacent genes. In other words, when the presence of a specific type of hormone is detected and binding occurs, this activates the receptor, and in medical (scientific) terms, the corresponding gene is either up-regulated or down-regulated, according to the normal function of the hormone. In more common terms, the activation of the receptor either switches the gene on or switches it off, depending on the normal purpose of that particular hormone.

Vitamin D is known to up-regulate many immune system defensive mechanisms.

Researchers have shown that vitamin D doesn't just provide a few immune system benefits here and there. It provides many benefits, which in many cases combine to present a formidable, broad-based set of defensive tools for dealing with specific health issues, by altering the expression of many genes that are associated with those issues.

In other words vitamin D is capable of turning certain genes on, and turning certain genes off, in order to assist the immune system in performing it's duties effectively. Since it appears that much more research has been done on the association of vitamin D and cancer, than on the association of vitamin D and AI diseases, let's explore this gene switching ability by considering some of the ways that vitamin D can inhibit the development of cancer cells.[16]

It has been well-established that $1,25(OH)_2D3$ expresses genes that interfere with the progress of cancer cell development cycles and promote apoptosis (to identify and destroy cancer cells). Other gene function alterations are triggered to cause weakened cellular adhesion, and to interfere with certain cancer cell immune functions. Genes that control internal cell communications and communications between cells are affected, resulting in compromised cancer cell communications. And numerous genes that affect the ability of cancer cells to reproduce and grow are controlled by 1,25(OH)$_2$D3.

Cancer cells utilize a process known as angiogenesis to create and develop expanded systems of new blood vessels that are capable of increasing the delivery of nutrients so that growth and development of new cancer cells can be expedited. This appears to be a primary mechanism that allows cancer to develop and spread so rapidly in many cases. By it's actions on certain genes, 1,25(OH)$_2$D3 helps to suppress the angiogenesis that supports rapid cancer growth, and other genes reduce the ability of cancer cells to spread to other areas of the body.[17] Vanoirbeek et al., (2011) concluded that, "Treatment with 1,25(OH)2D3 or its analogs, either alone or in combination with active anti-cancer drugs, may be able to prevent cancer initiation and/or delay cancer progression" (p. 599).

It's very, very likely that vitamin D provides a similar multifaceted approach to the control and prevention of autoimmune diseases also, because researchers have discovered that there is an important immune-related link between cancer and certain autoimmune diseases. Consider myasthenia gravis (MG), for example. MG is a serious muscle disease caused by the degrading or loss of autonomic nervous system control. It can cause many serious health problems, including breathing difficulties, heart rate control, the ability to swallow food, the ability to walk, and many other issues that are normally automatically controlled by our autonomic nervous system.

An important link between cancer and autoimmune disease has been found in a protein known as survivin.

While survivin is highly expressed in fetal tissue during development, it's normally absent from adult tissue.[18] Very recently, researchers have discovered that the T-cell lymphocytes that are responsible for the inflammation that causes MG, contain survivin.[19] Survivin is well known to cancer researchers, because it is one of the proteins known as "inhibitors of apoptosis proteins" (IAPs). In medical circles, survivin is also known as baculoviral inhibitor of apoptosis repeat-containing 5 (BIRC5). In humans, it's encoded by the BIRC5 gene.

As the descriptive name suggests, these proteins share the distinction of being able to inhibit programmed cell death. Obviously this implies that IAPs are capable of preventing the immune system from destroying cells that are protected by IAPs, and this technique is a primary survival tool used by cancer cells.

So now we can see that the inability of the immune system to clear the debris at inflammation sites may not be simply due to an overwhelming accumulation of debris because of chronic inflammation. The primary cause of the interrupted healing process may be due to the inability of the immune system to proceed with the process of apoptosis (due to the presence of inflammatory T-cells protected by survivin, or possibly another inhibitor of apoptosis protein). If these T-cells cannot be stopped by the immune system (by apoptosis) from continuing to inflame surrounding cells, then existing debris cannot be properly disposed of so that the damaged cells in the area can be replaced with new, healthy cells.

Kusner, Ciesielski, Marx, Kaminski, and Fenstermaker (2014) discovered that the autoreactive lymphocytes of myasthenia gravis patients contain the IAP survivin, whereas the lymphocytes of normal individuals do not.[20] Hopefully, this will lead to the development of new treatment methods for myasthenia gravis, but of equal importance is the possibility that it may lead to breakthroughs in treatment methods for autoimmune diseases in general.

How does the body normally prevent autoimmune reactions from developing?

The body has a specialized organ designed to train immature T-cell lymphocytes to locate and destroy antigens and other foreign invaders that might have the potential to harm us. This organ is known as the thymus. Immature progenitor cells, known as thymocytes are converted into T-cells, and by the use of a random generation process they are each individually configured to attack a specific (unique) antigen, and to ignore everything else. In order to ensure that they will not attack the body's own tissues (which by definition would be an autoimmune type reaction), the thymus is programmed to mark any cells that display a tendency to attack the body's own tissues (self) for apoptosis, so that they will be destroyed rather than to be allowed to be added to the arsenal of defensive tools available to the immune system for fighting disease.

But the thymus becomes less effective as we age.

We know from research studies that the thymus is most active when we are young, and it's function seems to peak about the time that we reach puberty. Beyond that point, the organ typically becomes less active, and it eventually loses much of it's functionality as we continue to age. Patel and Taub (2009) explored this issue and noted that various neuropeptides, hormones, and growth factors can combine with the effects of stress and increasing age to adversely influence the function of the thymus.[21]

But because of survivin, certain corrupt T-cells are able to escape apoptosis in the thymus.

Kusner, Ciesielski, Marx, Kaminski, and Fenstermaker (2014) discovered that the thymus of patients who had myasthenia gravis contained large numbers of cells that tested positive for survivin, but patients who were treated with corticosteroids had far fewer survivin-positive cells in their thymus. This discovery is of great interest, since Hidalgo, Deeb, Pike, Johnson, and Trump, (2011) showed that glucocorticoids increase the expression of vitamin D receptors, thereby increasing the effectiveness of vitamin D.[22] And of course glucocorticoids are a type of corticosteroid, so that means that corticosteroids help to express VDRs, and to enhance the effectiveness of vitamin D.

73

So I'll pose an academic question here, "Could this possibly be the primary mechanism by which corticosteroids work to suppress inflammation?"

Corticosteroids are widely prescribed to treat IBDs, rheumatoid arthritis, and other autoimmune diseases and inflammation-driven issues. It was previously thought that corticosteroids are effective for controlling inflammation because they suppress mast cell numbers and mast cell degranulation. But now we know that this is the domain of vitamin D and the vitamin D receptors.

Could it be that a synergistic effect with vitamin D might be the sole reason why corticosteroids are so effective at reducing inflammation? As you probably recall, a synergistic effect is one in which a combination of 2 or more chemical agents produces a stronger effect than the sum of the individual effects of the 2 substances when acting independently. Hopefully, a research group somewhere in the world will be curious enough (and able to find the necessary funding) to explore this and either verify it or disprove it. But in the meantime, my gut feeling is that corticosteroids probably suppress inflammation by expressing VDRs, thus exploiting vitamin D to actually provide the mechanism by which the inflammation is suppressed.

My position is supported by the fact that it is well known that corticosteroids deplete supplies of vitamin D in the body.[23] Obviously if corticosteroids promote the expression of VDRs, then this action would expedite increased utilization of available supples of vitamin D, resulting in depleted supples as the vitamin D is used to suppress the inflammation.

So if this turns out to be true, then the obvious question is, "Will corticosteroid treatments be modified in the future?"

Instead of using corticosteroids to treat inflammation, will the emphasis shift toward using corticosteroids as a means of enhancing the inflammation-fighting qualities of vitamin D? Probably not, if the pharmaceutical companies have their way, because that might cost them billions of dollars worth of lost sales of expensive drugs in the long run.

Of course more importantly, it might help to spare many thousands of patients from suffering from the often Draconian side effects so common with the use of corticosteroids. By optimizing (minimizing) corticosteroid dosages in order to target optimum vitamin D utilization, side effect risks could be significantly reduced.

But of course all of this remains to be verified by future research. And it's a safe bet that the giant pharmaceutical companies will fight this tooth and nail, since they will obviously not be interested in entertaining any thoughts about options that might result in potential lost sales revenue. And since most research is funded by the pharmaceutical companies, finding funding for such research may turn out to be quite a formidable task. Most research labs have a very close dependency on their primary sources of funding, so they might be very reluctant to take on a project that might alienate their traditional sources of support.

In view of the current research funding environment, it's probably a safe bet that research on this concept is not likely to see much activity in the near future. And as always, it will be the consumers (patients) who will suffer as a result of the current trend for research to promote the use of more drugs, and increasingly expensive drugs, rather than to pursue safe, inexpensive treatments based on diet changes or the use of supplements to prevent disease so that intervention with prescription drugs might be minimized or eliminated altogether.

A similar problem exists with certain B-cells.

Returning our attention to the myasthenia gravis research data cited earlier, the same researchers (Kusner, Ciesielski, Marx, Kaminski, & Fenstermaker, 2014) also found that myasthenia gravis patients had B-cells that tested positive for survivin. B lymphocytes mature in bone marrow, and when mature, their primary functions are to produce antibodies that target specific antigens, act as antigen-presenting cells, and to develop into memory B-cells after being activated by an antigen, as an important part of the adaptive immune system.

Similar to T-cells, B-cells are not allowed to mature and enter the immune system arsenal if they display any tendency to react to "self". Normally, any B-cells that show autoreactive characteristics are destroyed before they are allowed to mature and leave bone marrow.

But somehow, some or all of both types of corrupt cells (both T-cells and B-cells that display autoreactive capabilities) manage to escape apoptosis, and become mature, functional cells. They apparently evade the process of apoptosis by means of the expression of survivin. The unanswered question of course is, "How do they manage to express survivin?"

Survivin has also been associated with rheumatoid arthritis and multiple sclerosis.

Researchers (Bokarewa, Lindblad, Bokarew, and Tarkowski, 2005) have previously verified that survivin is present in the synovial tissue of severely-affected joints of rheumatoid arthritis patients.[24] And other research done by Hebb et al. (2008) found elevated levels of survivin in T-cells and brain tissue of multiple sclerosis patients.[25]

So it appears that survivin is a common thread among AI diseases. But interestingly, Bokarewa, Lindblad, Bokarew, and Tarkowski, (2005) found that high levels of anti-survivin antibodies appear to be a marker of less severe disease. What does that suggest? It implies that when the immune system is properly activated, in other words when adequate levels of vitamin D receptors are expressed (as described by the research previously discussed in this chapter), then the capacity of the disease to damage tissue (and to cause clinical symptoms) is significantly down-regulated.

That observation is supported by research data published by Li et al. (2004) showing that the mechanism by which vitamin D is able to inhibit the growth of cancer cells and induce apoptosis, is at least partially dependent upon the ability of vitamin D to down-regulate survivin.[26]

Vitamin D works synergistically with testosterone to down-regulate survivin.

Research data related to prostate cancer shows that while testosterone has the capacity to slightly down-regulate the expression of survivin, and vitamin D also has that capability, the combination of the 2 hormones creates a very synergistic down-regulation of the BIRC5 gene, resulting in a significantly-reduced level of survivin in prostate cancer patients (Wang, Chatterjee, Chittur, Welsh, & Tenniswood, 2011).[27]

But doesn't all this prove that the immune system becomes corrupt (contrary to my original claim)?

I stated back in chapter 1 that despite the medical community opinion that autoimmunity requires a corrupt immune system, my own interpretation disagrees with that claim. And in my opinion, the research evidence described above supports my position, rather than to contradict it.

Why? Because the basic problem that creates an environment that can lead up to the escape of corrupt T-cells and B-cells is a deficiency of vitamin D. That is something over which the immune system has absolutely no control.

Exactly How Does Vitamin D Deficiency Lead to Autoimmune Disease?

Instead, it's something that falls under out own personal responsibility. It's our duty as the owner of our body to keep it properly supplied with the fuel that it needs so that it can operate properly. We wouldn't expect our automobile to operate properly without an adequate supply of the correct fuel, so why would we expect our immune system, or any other part of our body to be able to perform optimally if we fail to supply the fuel that it needs.

It's not like the immune system suddenly goes berserk and turns on the body. That doesn't happen. Just as our heart and our circulatory system, and the process by which cells are supplied with nutrients, require at least a certain minimum level of electrolytes in order to function correctly, the immune system has to have an adequate supply of vitamin D if it is to perform optimally. If it fails to perform up to standard, it's not because it has become corrupt, but because it is being starved for an essential hormone.

As long as we do not allow our body to become starved for vitamin D, those autoreactive cells will be destroyed by the immune system, just as nature intended. They will be removed from the system before they can cause any harm.

Remember that this is a normal function of the immune system. Therefore the immune system will be prevented from becoming corrupted, as long as it is allowed to function normally. Clearly, the basic problem is not a defective immune system — it's a problem of starving our immune system for a vital hormone, namely vitamin D.

Will the discovery of a synergistic effect between vitamin D and testosterone affect the way that prostate cancer is treated in the future?

Interestingly, traditional prostate cancer treatments typically include measures to lower testosterone levels in the body (called androgen deprivation therapy [ADT] or androgen suppression therapy), because conventional medical wisdom says that testosterone promotes cancer growth. It will be interesting to see how long it takes for these well-established treatment practices to be altered to incorporate the use of vitamin D in order to induce a synergistic effect with testosterone to suppress survivin levels in prostate cancer patients. Not only should this combination help to prevent the development of prostate cancer, but with survivin suppressed, the immune system should be able to kill existing cancer cells as part of its normal functionality.

As we have seen, many researchers have provided extensive data to show that the combination of vitamin D and vitamin D receptors is necessary in order to accomplish these powerful effects to suppress and prevent disease. And while it's clear that we can increase our vitamin D level simply by either increasing our skin exposure to sunlight in areas of the world where this is effective, or by increasing our supplemental oral vitamin D intake, it's not so clear how we can boost our supply of vitamin D receptors.

So how do we increase our VDR count?

Fortunately, some very recent research sheds some light on this important topic. Endothelial dysfunction is a common problem associated with many cardiovascular issues. The endothelium is the medical term for the inner lining of blood vessels, and endothelial dysfunction refers to an inability of blood vessels to function normally. This condition is typically associated with inflammation, and it normally precedes the development of atherosclerosis. With endothelial dysfunction, blood vessels are unable to adequately dilate as needed, in order to properly accommodate changes in blood pressure, and blood flow rates, thus leading to hypertension and other related issues.

But Zhong, Gu, Gu, Groome, Sun, and Wang. (2014) discovered that the active form of vitamin D (1,25[OH]$_2$D3) is capable of promoting an increase in VDR expression, and to add credibility to it's effectiveness, the increase occurs in a dose-and time-dependent manner.[28] In addition, the researchers discovered that if they starved endothelial cells for oxygen, in order to introduce oxidative stress, this would suppress the number of VDRs. But if adequate 1,25(OH)$_2$D3 were available, the depletion of VDR numbers was prevented. Needless to say, such a powerful antioxidant effect is extremely impressive.

Now clearly this research was confined specifically to endothelial cells, so we can't claim that this proves that the findings apply in other situations, but it doesn't take a rocket scientist to recognize that there is a very good chance that this effect will probably apply in other situations where vitamin D has already been

81

shown to produce dramatic health-enhancing and disease-preventing benefits. Hopefully research to confirm this will soon follow.

Note that this phenomenon (based on the expression of survivin) may not be the only immune system mechanism by which autoimmune reactions may manage to escape the built-in checks and balances that are designed to prevent AI reactions, but it certainly appears to be one that could be significant enough to cause serious AI issues. And at this point, this appears to be the only possibility that researchers have been able to identify in numerous AI syndromes, and more than a few groups of researchers have verified the same basic observations. This strongly supports the science behind the discovery.

So now we understand why vitamin D deficiency leads to autoimmune disease. And we also understand how an adequate blood level of vitamin D can play a major role in preventing the development of autoimmune disease and many other health issues.

Summary

Recent research has shown that similar to cancer, certain autoreactive T-cells and B-cells may be able to escape apoptosis by utilizing the inappropriate expression of an inhibitor of apoptosis protein known as survivin. As a result, they are able to escape being destroyed by the immune system, resulting in their ability to not only promote, but to perpetuate inflammation in various organs and joints. This is the essence of autoimmunity.

Exactly How Does Vitamin D Deficiency Lead to Autoimmune Disease?

Furthermore, research shows that this condition of autoreactivity appears to be caused by a vitamin D deficiency. Fortunately there are plenty of research data available to show that a primary key to preventing the development of autoimmune disease is to insure that at least a sufficient blood level of vitamin D is always available. It may be as simple as that, for many of us.

Chapter 6

Should We Be Taking a Vitamin D Supplement?

Research shows that food is not a reliable source of vitamin D in most cases.

The form of vitamin D that we are always initially exposed to is the inactive form, whether it be produced in our own body by the action of ultraviolet-B rays in sunlight on a derivative of cholesterol (known as 7-dehydrocholesterol) at the surface of our skin, or from sources of vitamin D in our food, or from an oral vitamin D supplement. But before the cells of our body can utilize it, most of the vitamin D must be converted to the active form, and this conversion mostly takes place in a process that begins in the liver and is completed in the kidneys.

I use the term "mostly" because there are other locations where minor amounts of vitamin D are converted into the active form. For example, in the previous chapter we discussed how mast cells are capable of converting vitamin D into the active form for their own purposes. But as we also learned in the previous chapter, most of the conversion of vitamin D into the active form begins in the liver and the process is completed in the kidneys.

Despite the claims of government authorities and many food "experts" that attempt to promote food as a viable source of vitamin D, according to the Vitamin D Council, it is very unlikely that most people would be able to get their vitamin D needs from their diet.[1] So that leaves exposure to sunlight, and vitamin D oral supplements as the only truly practical sources of vitamin D for most of us. Note that while it is impossible to acquire toxic levels of vitamin D from sunlight exposure, it is certainly possible to reach toxic blood levels of vitamin D by means of medium-term or long-term use of relatively high daily doses of supplemental vitamin D. We will explore that risk in more detail later in this chapter.

The best source of vitamin D is sunlight on our skin.

In order to make vitamin D naturally, our skin must be exposed to an adequate amount of sunlight for an adequate length of time, and since approximately 48 hours is required for the chemical process to be completed after it is initiated by the sun exposure, we must refrain from washing away the oily substance on our skin that contains the intermediate stage chemicals, or we will wash away the vitamin D before it is completely created, and before most of it becomes available to be absorbed into our skin. Light rinsing with plain water may not remove all of these intermediate substances, but scrubbing with soap and water will certainly remove them and terminate the vitamin D production process prematurely.

In the summer, at lower latitudes (closer to the equator), sun exposure requirements may be minimal, and only 10 or 15 minutes of exposure time may be necessary in order to generate more than enough vitamin D to supply our daily needs. But the amount of vitamin D produced will depend on a number of limiting conditions, which according to The Vitamin D Council, include (but are not limited to) factors such as:[1]

> 1. Time of day – skin exposure in the middle of the day is much more productive than at other times of the day.
>
> 2. Location – more sunlight is available closer to the equator, so the skin can produce more vitamin D in less time.
>
> 3. Skin pigmentation – darker skins take longer to produce vitamin D than light-colored skins when exposed to an equal amount of sunlight.
>
> 4. Exposed surface area of skin – a larger exposed surface area will obviously lead to higher vitamin D production rates than smaller exposed areas of skin.
>
> 5. Our age — as we age, our skin becomes less efficient at producing vitamin D.

6. Use of sunscreen — obviously sunscreen blocks much (in many situations, most to virtually all) of the potential vitamin D production that might otherwise be available.

7. Altitude — the higher the altitude, the more intense the sunlight, and therefore the greater the potential for producing vitamin D.

8. Clouds — clouds scatter light, which reduces the amount of sunlight passing through, and therefore they tend to reduce the amount to vitamin D that we may be able to produce on a cloudy day.

9. Air pollution — similar to clouds, air pollution tends to scatter, reflect, and absorb ultraviolet B light, which reduces our ability to produce vitamin D when air pollution is at a significant level.

10. Glass — glass blocks ultraviolet B light, which will prevent our skin from being able to produce vitamin D if there is a glass surface between our skin and the sun.

So obviously, determining the amount of vitamin D that we may be getting from the sun, turns out to be quite complicated. Depending on all of the limiting factors listed above, it's easily possible to produce 10,000–25,000 IU of vitamin D during a session of sun exposure under optimum conditions. But under the poorest conditions, the amount of vitamin D produced might range down to virtually nothing. And if that happens to be our situation, then we must turn to supplements in order to maintain an adequate level of vitamin D in our body.

If we take supplemental vitamin D, how much should we take?

That's the 64 dollar question. Note that in some countries, vitamin D is listed in micrograms (mcg). It's easy to convert the amounts, since 1 mcg = 40 IU. Therefore, 25 mcg of vitamin D would be equal to 1,000 IU of vitamin D.

Unfortunately it's not easy to decide how much vitamin D to take, because "official" guidelines are all over the place. For example, the official government source, the Institute of Medicine, says that a daily estimated average requirement (EAR) of 400 IU of vitamin D is adequate for the average adult. They go on to specify a recommended dietary allowance (RDA) of 600 IU up until the age of 70, and 800 IU beyond that age. They show 4,000 IU as the tolerable upper intake level (UL), implying that no one should ever take more than 4,000 IU as a daily dose.

And if you believe that those recommendations are valid after reading the research articles that are cited in the previous chapters, you have a lot more faith in the published government guidelines than I have. Obviously many experts disagree with those recommendations. For example, the Endocrine Practice Guidelines Committee of the Endocrine Society recommends 1,500–2,000 IU as a daily requirement for adults, and considers 10,000 IU to be the upper limit.[2]

Vitamin D Deficiency and Autoimmune Disease

According to the Vitamin D Council, the average daily usage level for vitamin D is around 5,000 IU. In other words, 5,000 IU is considered to be the approximate amount of vitamin D that an average individual might use each day, so it seems logical that we should take in at least 5,000 IU each day, from all sources, on the average. If we get sufficient sun exposure, and we live close enough to the equator, then the sun may provide enough vitamin D to supply our needs.

But if that doesn't apply to our situation, then we will need additional vitamin D, either from our food, or from a supplement, or we may be likely to eventually develop a deficiency. And as we previously noted, most of us are not likely to be successful in acquiring an adequate amount of vitamin D from our diet, though we would probably be able to get a percentage of our needs from our food.

Of course vitamin D needs can vary widely, depending on individual characteristics. As we have already seen, certain autoimmune diseases tend to deplete our body's supply of vitamin D, and those same diseases tend to inhibit the absorption of vitamin D. So obviously if we have such a condition, then we may need to take significantly more supplemental vitamin D than someone who does not have any autoimmune issues for example, or we will have a higher risk of developing a vitamin D deficiency, which can make us vulnerable to the development of additional autoimmune diseases. And anyone using certain medications such as corticosteroids and bisphosphonates will have a need for additional vitamin D.

Therefore it may be prudent to have our vitamin D level tested occasionally, especially if we have reason to believe that it may not be in the normal range. Or if we have been taking an increased dose of supplemental vitamin D in order to raise our blood level of vitamin D, it is usually a good plan to have the level checked after several months, and then reassess our supplement dosage based on the test results.

If for any reason your doctor is not willing to order a vitamin D test for you, anyone can order a blood spot test for vitamin D on the Internet, from the lab at the following URL. I have compared the results of these tests with the results provided by the lab my own doctor uses, and as long as the blood draws are made no more than a day or so apart, the results have been identical. And in case you're wondering — no, I have no business affiliation with this lab other than as a satisfied customer.

https://store.zrtlab.com/index.php/blood-spot-testing

Is it possible to take too much vitamin D?

While the formation of vitamin D from sun exposure cannot cause a toxic overdose condition, as we are well aware, it's certainly possible to reach a toxic condition by taking high doses of a vitamin D supplement for an extended period of time. It's necessary to use common sense when taking any type of vitamin supplements. In general, someone taking 5,000 IU of vitamin D daily for example, may or may not gradually increase their blood level of 25(OH)D, but they are not likely to ever reach a toxic condition at that dosage rate. By contrast, someone who takes 40,000 IU each day for an extended period, will almost surely reach a toxic condition after a few months of taking such a high dose. In between these extremes lies a broad gray area.

Too much vitamin D tends to cause excessive calcium absorption, so high blood levels of vitamin D can lead to a dangerous condition known as hypercalcemia. To date, it appears that all known cases of vitamin D toxicity associated with hypercalcemia have been a result of extended periods of daily vitamin D intakes of over 40,000 IU.[3] Therefore, in cases where vitamin D deficiency or insufficiency needs to be corrected, a daily dosage in the range of 5,000–10,000 IU for several weeks or so would not seem unreasonable, provided that the blood level is tested occasionally in order to monitor the progress of the treatment. Beyond that though, higher doses taken for extended periods of time can be risky.

Taking for example, 15,000–20,000 IU daily for a few weeks probably would not cause any problems, but taking that much for several months could be asking for trouble. Unfortunately the medical literature is severely lacking when it comes to specific information on vitamin D toxicity. It mostly consists of case studies and speculation. But since there's really nothing to be gained by taking megadoses, why take a chance on overdoing it? If we keep the supplementation rates within common sense limits, then we should have nothing to worry about.

Too much vitamin D can cause gastrointestinal symptoms such as nausea and vomiting. Other symptoms can include high blood pressure, excessive production of urine, weakness, anxiety, nervousness, and itching.

While experts warn us about the risks of vitamin D toxicity, the reality is that most vitamin D toxicity cases have been caused by manufacturing or industrial accidents, because it takes a heck of a lot of supplemental vitamin D, for a relatively long period of time, to cause a toxic condition — so much that it's highly unlikely that most individuals who have at least a rudimentary understanding of the risks involved with taking supplemental vitamin D would ever accidentally or intentionally use that much.

If a toxic level of vitamin D should develop, the usual treatment is to just stop taking the supplement and limit calcium intake. If hypercalcemia is at a severe level, serum calcium levels can be reduced by taking a corticosteroid.[4]

How do we go about determining a good starting dose?

One of the most trusted Internet sources of medical information that's widely used by physicians is Medscape.com. Medscape has an excellent article that provides some insight into how much increase in a patient's vitamin D blood level can be expected if certain specific dosages of supplemental vitamin D are taken daily for 2 or 3 months. Some of the examples listed in the article are:[5]

- *400 IU (10 mcg) per day increases vitamin D blood levels 4 ng/ml (10 nmol/L).*

- *500 IU (12.5 mcg) per day increases vitamin D blood levels 5 ng/ml (12.5 nmol/L).*

Vitamin D Deficiency and Autoimmune Disease

- *800 IU (20 mcg) per day increases vitamin D blood levels 8 ng/ml (20 nmol/L).*

- *1000 IU (25 mcg) per day increases vitamin D blood levels 10 ng/ml (25 nmol/L).*

- *2000 IU (50 mcg) per day increases vitamin D blood levels 20 ng/ml (50 nmol/L).*

So based on these guidelines, if we were to take the daily dosage recommended by the government's Institute of Medicine (400 IU), then at the end of several months we would be likely to have increased our blood level of vitamin D by only about 4 ng/ml (10 nmol/l). Obviously if we have a vitamin D deficiency, that's not going to provide any significant benefit, especially if we have a health issue such as an autoimmune disease that's imposing increased demands upon our vitamin D reserves.

Also note that responses to supplemental vitamin D will vary by the individual. These guidelines appear to be recommended for someone who has a vitamin D deficiency. Age, existing health issues, and our current vitamin D blood level will affect how well we will respond to any supplemental treatment program. The lower our current vitamin D blood level, the greater our response will be to any given supplemental dosage.

Conversely, the higher our current vitamin D level, the smaller our gain will be. Therefore if we have a specific goal in mind, (for example, maybe we want to raise our level by 20 ng/ml [50 nmol/l]), and our current vitamin D blood level is at a normal (sufficient) level or above, a larger supplemental dose than suggested by these guidelines will probably be necessary in order to reach that goal within a reasonable amount of time (several months).

And after we manage to reach a higher blood level of vitamin D that meets our goal, then we will find it necessary to continue to take an appropriate maintenance dose of vitamin D in order to maintain that level. Otherwise our vitamin D level will slowly decline back to where it was before we began taking a vitamin D supplement. The size of the maintenance dose will obviously be smaller than the dose that we used to increase the level, but the higher the blood level of vitamin D that we wish to maintain, the higher the dose will need to be. And of course having an active IBD for example, would mean that a higher supplemental maintenance dose would be required.

We may need to allow for the effects of certain medications.

Remember that medical treatments that involve either a corticosteroid or a bisphosphonate can significantly lower one's available vitamin D reserves (requiring additional supplemental vitamin D in order to avoid becoming deficient). And as we get older, we typically need more supplemental vitamin D in order to maintain a safe blood level (because we tend to absorb vitamin D less efficiently as we age).

These of course are very likely common reasons why the risk of developing autoimmune disease increases significantly as we get older, because physicians typically don't remind us that we may need additional vitamin D. They may not even be aware of an increased need. In fact, it seems that vitamin D, as important as it is for long-term health, is often not even on most doctors' radar. I have a hunch that this will change as they become more aware of recent research, and they see for themselves the dramatic health improvements that vitamin D can bring in many cases.

But are the official guidelines for a "sufficient" vitamin D level actually sufficient?

The kicker is that levels of serum vitamin D claimed to be "sufficient" by many sources (particularly those affiliated with the government), are actually only sufficient to prevent the development of rickets in the majority of cases. Looking beyond that limited level of sufficiency, researchers have shown that higher average blood levels of vitamin D will effectively help to reduce the incidence of many common diseases in the general population.

In fact it has been shown that improved prevention of certain specific diseases are associated with certain respective vitamin D levels. In other words, the concept of "vitamin D sufficiency" is not a one-size-fits-all situation. The relationship between vitamin D levels and improved disease resistance for specific diseases is somewhat complex, but data that can be used as guidelines are available. Fortunately, a convenient chart showing some of those relationships has been compiled by the Grassroots Health organization, and it can be viewed on the Internet at this URL:[6]

Should We Be Taking a Vitamin D Supplement?

http://www.grassrootshealth.net/media/download/disease_incid
ence_prev_chart_032310.pdf

Note that for example, according to that chart, compared with a baseline serum vitamin D level of 25 ng/ml (62 nmol/l), a 25(OH)D level of 34 ng/ml (85 nmol/l) is associated with a 30 % reduction in breast cancer incidence. At a 25(OH)D level of 50 ng/ml (125 nmol/l), the projected reduction in the incidence of breast cancer is a very impressive 83 %.

As another example from that chart, consider Type 1 diabetes. The chart shows that compared with a baseline 25(OH)D level of 25 ng/ml (62 nmol/l), a vitamin D blood level of 36 ng/ml (90 nmol/l) is associated with a 25 % reduction in incidence, whereas a 25(OH)D level of 52 ng/ml (130 nmol/l) is associated with a 66 % reduction in the incidence of Type 1 diabetes.

The equivalent reductions in incidence for multiple sclerosis are 33 % at a serum vitamin D level of 44 ng/ml (110 nmol/l), a known reduction of 46 % at 50 ng;/ml, and a projected 54 % reduction at a 25(OH)D level of 54 ng/ml (135 nmol/l). Again, these reductions are based on a comparison with a baseline vitamin D serum level of 25 ng/ml (62 nmol/l).

There currently seems to be a considerable amount of interest in pursuing research in this area. And as more data become available to fill in the gaps, that information will continue to advance our understanding of how vitamin D prevents autoimmune disease, and how it manages to provide so many other health benefits. This is an exciting period of time to be alive, because many of the long-held (incorrect) medical assumptions about major health issues, and particularly the effects of diet on health, are beginning to fall by the wayside, as the truth finally becomes evident.

Summary

While the exposure of our skin to sunlight is always the best way to meet our vitamin D needs, if that option is not available, or not adequate, then oral vitamin D supplements are a practical alternative. As is the case with any vitamin supplements, we have to use common sense and not take excessively large doses for extended periods of time, because that can possibly lead to a condition of toxic overdose.

Determining our own personal "ideal" vitamin D level requires some thought, since it may depend on our lifestyle, our environment, and any existing health issues that we may already have. Actually achieving that level can be somewhat complex, and is best accomplished by consulting with one's primary care practitioner in order to coordinate testing and establishing trial dosages of vitamin D. But if it becomes obvious that our doctor doesn't appear to understand the importance of maintaining an adequate level of vitamin D that will serve us well, it's comforting to remember that it's possible to order the tests that are needed online, so that we don't have to wonder if our vitamin D level is sufficient to meet our needs.

It's worth noting that while the low vitamin D supplementation rates recommended by most official government guidelines are sufficient for preventing such easy-to-prevent diseases as rickets, research shows that higher blood levels of vitamin will effective-ly lower the statistical risk of developing many other diseases. For certain types of cancer and major autoimmune diseases, higher vitamin D levels have been associated with significantly lower odds of developing those diseases.

References

Chapter 1

How Autoimmune Disease Develops

1. Rosea, N. R., & Bona, C. (1993). Defining criteria for autoimmune diseases (Witebsky's postulates revisited). *Immunology Today, 14*(9), 426–430. Retrieved from http://www.ncbi.nlm.nih.gov/pubmed/8216719

2. Davis, E. (2008). USDA food pyramid history. [Web log message]. Retrieved from http://www.healthy-eating-politics.com/usda-food-pyramid.html

3. Fasano, A. (2012). Leaky gut and autoimmune diseases. *Clinical Reviews in Allergy and Immunology, 42*(1), 71–78. doi:10.1007/s12016-011-8291-x

4. Persky, W. (2012). *Microscopic Colitis*. Bartlett, TX: Persky Farms

Chapter 2

The Conditions Necessary for Healing to Occur

1. Rubio-Tapia, A., Rahim, M. W., See, J. A., Lahr, B. D., Tsung-Teh Wu, T-T., & Murray, J. A. (2010). Mucosal recovery and mortality in adults with celiac disease after treatment with a gluten-free diet. *The American Journal of Gastroenterology, 105*(1), 1,412–1,420. doi:10.1038/ajg.2010.10

2. Bardella, M. T., Velio, P., Cesana, B. M., Prampolini, L., Casella, G., Di Bella, C., . . . Villanacci, V. (2007). Coeliac disease: A histological follow-up study. *Histopathology, 50*(4), 465–471. Retrieved from
http://www.ingentaconnect.com/content/bsc/histo/2007/00000050/00000004/art00008

Chapter 3

Vitamin D Deficiency Has Been Shown to Be Linked With Many Autoimmune Diseases

1. Bozkurt, N. C., Karbek, B., Ucan, B., Sahin, M., Cakal, E., Ozbek, M., & Delibasi, T. (2013). The association between severity of vitamin D deficiency and Hashimoto's thyroiditis. *En-*

Vitamin D Deficiency Has Been Shown to Be Linked With Many Autoimmune Diseases

docrine Practice, 21, 1–14. Advance online publication. Retrieved from http://www.ncbi.nlm.nih.gov/pubmed/23337162

2. Syed, M. A., Barinas-Mitchell, E., Pietropaolo, S. L., Zhang, Y. J., Henderson, T. S., Kelley, D. E., . . . Pietropaolo, M. (2002). Is type 2 diabetes a chronic inflammatory/autoimmune disease? *Diabetes, Nutrition & Metabolism, 15*(2), 68–83. Retrieved from http://www.ncbi.nlm.nih.gov/pubmed/12059095

3. Maugh II, T. H. (2011, April 18). Type 2 diabetes, like type 1, may be an autoimmune disease, researchers say. *Los Angeles Times*. Retrieved from http://articles.latimes.com/2011/apr/18/news/la-heb-diabetes-au-toimmune-04182011

4. Gardner, A. (2013, February 20). 1 in 8 Americans diagnosed with type 2 diabetes: Poll. [Web log message]. Retrieved from http://consumer.healthday.com/Article.asp?AID=673579

5. Munger, K. L., Levin, L. I., Massa, J., Horst, R., Orban, T., & Ascherio, A. (2012). Preclinical serum 25-hydroxyvitamin D levels and risk of type 1 diabetes in a cohort of US military personnel. *American Journal of Epidemiology, 177*(5), 411–419. doi:10.1093/aje/kws243

6. Walsh, N. (2013, February 4). Arthritis: Sun's rays may cut risk in women. [Web log message]. Retrieved from http://www.med-pagetoday.com/Rheumatology/Arthritis/37187

7. Cutolo, M., Otsa, K., Laas, K., Yprus, M., Lehtme, R., Secchi, M. E., . . . Seriolo, B. (2006). Circannual vitamin d serum levels and disease activity in rheumatoid arthritis: Northern versus Southern Europe. *Clinical and Experimental Rheumatology*, 24(6), 702–704. Retrieved from http://www.ncbi.nlm.nih.gov/pubmed/17207389

8. Derakhshandi, H., Etemadifar, M., Feizi, A., Abtahi, S. H., Minagar, A., Abtahi, M. A., . . . Tabrizi, N. (2013). Preventive effect of vitamin D3 supplementation on conversion of optic neuritis to clinically definite multiple sclerosis: a double blind, randomized, placebo-controlled pilot clinical trial. *Acta Neurologica Belgica*, 113(3), 257–263. doi:10.1007/s13760-012-0166-2

9. Mostafa, G. A., & AL-Ayadhi, L. Y. (2012). Reduced serum concentrations of 25-hydroxy vitamin D in children with autism: Relation to autoimmunity. *Journal of Neuroinflammation*, 9, 201 doi:10.1186/1742-2094-9-201

10. Mostafa, G. A., Al Shehab, A., & Fouad, N. R. (2010). Frequency of CD4+CD25high regulatory T cells in the peripheral blood of Egyptian children with autism. *Journal of Child Neurology*, 25(3), 328–335. doi:10.1177/0883073809339393

11. Lim, W. C., Hanauer, S. B., & Li, Y. C. (2005). Mechanisms of disease: Vitamin D and inflammatory bowel disease. *Nature Clinical Practice Gastroenterology & Hepatology*, 2(7), 308–315. Retrieved from http://www.ncbi.nlm.nih.gov/pubmed/16265284

12. Farraye, F. A., Nimitphong, H., Stucchi, A., Dendrinos, K., Boulanger, A. B., Vijjeswarapu, A., . . . Holick, M. F. (2011). Use of a novel vitamin D bioavailability test demonstrates that vitamin D absorption is decreased in patients with quiescent Crohn's disease. *Inflammatory Bowel Disease, 17*(10), 2,116–2,121. doi:10.1002/ibd.21595

Chapter 4

Many Non-Autoimmune Diseases Are Also Associated With Vitamin D Deficiency

1. Center to Reduce Cancer Health Disparities, (2013). 2013 Annual report to the nation on the status of cancer. *U.S. National Institutes of Health — National Cancer Institute.* [Web log message]. Retrieved from http://crchd.cancer.gov/news/report-nation_2013.html#Incidence

2. Huang, G-L., Yang, L., Su, M., Wang, S-K., Yin, H., Wang, J.-S., & Sun, G.-J. (2014). Vitamin D3 and beta-carotene deficiency is associated with risk of esophageal squamous cell carcinoma - Results of a case-control study in China. *Asian Pacific Journal of Cancer Prevention, 15*(2), 819–823. doi:10.7314/APJCP.2014.15.2.819

3. Mohr, S. B., Gorham, E. D., Kim, J., Hofflich, H., & Garland, C. F. (2014). Meta-analysis of vitamin D sufficiency for improving

survival of patients with breast cancer. *Anticancer Research,* 34(3), 1,163–1,166. Retrieved from www.ncbi.nlm.nih.gov/pubmed/24596354

4. Atkinson, M. A., Melamed, M, L., Kumar, J., Roy, C. N., Miller, E. R., Furth, S. L., & Fadrowski, J. J. (2014). Vitamin D, race, and risk for anemia in children. *Journal of Pediatrics, 164*(1), 153–158. doi:10.1016/j.jpeds.2013.08.060

5. Schroth, R. J., Lavelle, C., Tate, R., Bruce, S., Billings, R. J., & Moffatt, M. E. K. (2014). Prenatal vitamin D and dental caries in infants. *Pediatrics,* Online publication. doi:10.1542/peds.2013-2215

6. Gracious, B. L., Finucane, T. L., Friedman-Campbell, M., Messing, S., & Parkhurst, M. N. (2012). Vitamin D deficiency and psychotic features in mentally ill adolescents: A cross-sectional study. *BioMed Central Psychiatry, 12*(38). doi:10.1186/1471-244X-12-38

7. Massey, M. (2014, March 31). Vitamin D may help prevent Alzheimer's disease. *Daily Herald,* Online publication. Retrieved from http://www.dailyherald.com/article/20140331/entlife/140339966/

8. Anderson, P. (2012, September 28). Low vitamin D linked to Alzheimer's disease. *Medscape.* [Web log message]. Retrieved from http://www.medscape.com/viewarticle/771782

9. Staff. (2012, November 8). Vitamin D could hold vital key to arresting development of Alzheimer's disease. *ScienceDaily*. [Web log message]. Retrieved from http://www.sciencedaily.com/releases/2012/11/121108131452.htm

10. Derakhshandi, H., Etemadifar, M., Feizi, A., Abtahi, S. H., Minagar, A., Abtahi, M. A., . . . Tabrizi, N. (2013). Preventive effect of vitamin D3 supplementation on conversion of optic neuritis to clinically definite multiple sclerosis: a double blind, randomized, placebo-controlled pilot clinical trial. *Acta Neurologica Belgica, 113*(3), 257–263. doi:10.1007/s13760-012-0166-2

11. Carmeli, C., Donati, A., Antille, V., Viceic, D., Ghika, J., von Gunten, A., . . . Knyazeva, M. G. (2013). Demyelination in mild cognitive impairment suggests progression path to Alzheimer's disease. *PLoS ONE 8*(8), e72759. doi:10.1371/journal.pone.0072759

12. Annweiler, C., Rolland, Y., Schott, A. M., Blain, H., Vellas, B., & Beauchet, O. (2011). Serum vitamin D deficiency as a predictor of incident non-Alzheimer dementias: a 7-year longitudinal study. *Dementia and Geriatric Cognitive Disorders, 32*(4), 273–278. doi:10.1159/000334944

13. Littlejohns, T. J., Henley, W. E., Lang, I. A., Annweiler, C., Beauchet, O., Chaves, P. H. M., . . . David J. Llewellyn, D. J. (2014). Vitamin D and the risk of dementia and Alzheimer disease. *Neurology*. Advance online publication. doi:10.1212/WNL.0000000000000755

Vitamin D Deficiency and Autoimmune Disease

14. Holick, M. F., (2005). The vitamin D epidemic and its health consequences. *The Journal of Nutrition, 135*, 2,739S–2,748S. Retrieved from http://jn.nutrition.org/content/135/11/2739S.full.pdf

15. Cannell, J. (2013, February 1). Is vitamin D involved with balance? *The Vitamin D Council.* {Web log message]. Retrieved from https://www.vitamindcouncil.org/blog/is-vitamin-d-involved-with-balance/#

16. Ramagopalan, S. V., Heger, A., Berlanga, A. J., Maugeri, N. J., Lincoln, M. R., Burrell, A., . . . Knight, J. C. (2010). A ChIP-seq defined genome-wide map of vitamin D receptor binding: Associations with disease and evolution. *Genome Research 20*, 1,352–1,360. Advance online publication. doi:10.1101/gr.107920.110

17. Holick, M. F., Vitamin D: Importance in the prevention of cancers, type 1 diabetes, heart disease, and osteoporosis. *The American Journal of Clinical Nutrition, 79*(3), 362–371. Retrieved from http://ajcn.nutrition.org/content/79/3/362.long

18. Mercola, J. (2014, February 16). Epidemic of infantile rickets may have put thousands of innocent parents in jail for child abuse. *Mercola.com.* [Web log message] Retrieved from http://articles.mercola.com/sites/articles/archive/2014/02/16/infantile-rickets.aspx

19. Lindqvist, P. G., Epstein, E., Landin-Olsson, M., Ingvar, C., Nielsen, K., Stenbeck, M., & Olsson, H. (2014). Avoidance of sun exposure is a risk factor for all-cause mortality: Results from the

melanoma in Southern Sweden cohort. *Journal of Internal Medicine, 276*(1), 77–86. doi:10.1111/joim.12251

Chapter 5

Exactly How Does Vitamin D Deficiency Lead to Autoimmune Disease?

1. Gardiner, L. (2004). How new cells are made: Mitosis. [Web log message]. Windows to the Universe - *National Earth Science Teachers Association.* Retrieved from http://www.windows2universe.org/earth/Life/cell_mitosis.html

2. How are new cells made? *Cancer Research UK.* [Web log message]. Retrieved from http://www.cancerresearchuk.org/cancer-info/cancerandresearch/all-about-cancer/what-is-cancer/making-new-cells/where-do-cancer-cells-come-from

3. Mok, C. C., Birmingham, D. J., Leung, H. W., Hebert, L. A., Song, H., & Rovin, B. H. (2011). Vitamin D levels in Chinese patients with systemic lupus erythematosus: relationship with disease activity, vascular risk factors and atherosclerosis. *Rheumatology, 51*(4), 644–652.. doi:10.1093/rheumatology/ker212

4. Munoz, L. E., Schiller, M., Zhao, Y., Voll, R. E., Schett, G., & Herrmann, M. (2011). Do low vitamin D levels cause problems of

waste removal in patients with SLE? *Rheumatology, 51*(4), 585–587. doi:10.1093/rheumatology/ker334

5. Science Hack!, (1999). Crawling neutrophil chasing a bacterium. Educational Science Videos. Retrieved from http://science-hack.com/videos/view/I_xh-bkiv_c

6. Chandra, G., Selvaraj, P., Jawahar, M. S., Banurekha, V. V., & Narayanan, P. R. (2004). Effect of vitamin D3 on phagocytic potential of macrophages with live Mycobacterium tuberculosis and lymphoproliferative response in pulmonary tuberculosis. *Journal of Clinical Immunology, 24*(3), 249–257. Retrieved from http://www.ncbi.nlm.nih.gov/pubmed/15114055

7. Houghton, L. A., & Vieth, R. (2006). The case against ergocalciferol (vitamin D_2) as a vitamin supplement. *American Journal of Clinical Nutrition, 84*(4), 694–697. Retrieved from http://ajcn.nutrition.org/content/84/4/694.full

8. Ritterhouse, L. L., Crowe, S. R., Niewold, T. B., Kamen, D. L., Macwana, S. R., Roberts, V. C., . . . James, J. A. (2011). Vitamin D deficiency is associated with an increased autoimmune response in healthy individuals and in patients with systemic lupus erythematosus. *Annals of the Rheumatic Diseases, 70*, 1,569–1,574. doi:10.1136/ard.2010.148494

9. Ramagopalan, S. V., Heger, A., Berlanga, A. J., Maugeri, N. J., Lincoln, M. R., Burrell, A., . . . Knight, J. C. (2010). A ChIP-seq defined genome-wide map of vitamin D receptor binding: Associa-

tions with disease and evolution. *Genome Research 20*, 1,352–1,360. Advance online publication. doi:10.1101/gr.107920.110

10. Staff. (2011, June 24). Vitamin D. *National Institutes of Health Office of Dietary Supplements.* Retrieved from http://ods.od.nih.-gov/factsheets/VitaminD-HealthProfessional/

11. Yip, K. H., Kolesnikoff, N., Yu, C., Hauschild, N., Taing, H., Biggs L., . . . Grimbaldeston, M. A. (2014). Mechanisms of vitamin D3 metabolite repression of IgE-dependent mast cell activation. *The Journal of Allergy and Clinical Immunology, 133*(5), 1,356–1,364. doi:10.1016/j.jaci.2013.11.030

12. Baroni, E., Biffi, M., Benigni, F., Monno, A., Carlucci, D., Carmeliet, G., . . . D'Ambrosio, D. (2007). VDR-dependent regulation of mast cell maturation mediated by 1,25-dihydroxyvitamin D3. *Journal of Leukocyte Biology, 81*(1), 250–262. doi:10.1189/jlb.0506322

13 Discussion and Support Forum for Collagenous Colitis, Lymphocytic Colitis, Microscopic Colitis, Mastocytic Enterocolitis, and Related Issues. (2014). *perskyfarms.com.* Retrieved from http://www.perskyfarms.com/phpBB2/index.php

14. Kong, J., Zhang, Z., Musch, M. W., Ning, G., Sun, J., Hart, J., . . . Li, Y. C. (2008). Novel role of the vitamin D receptor in maintaining the integrity of the intestinal mucosal barrier. *American Journal of Physiology - Gastrointestinal and Liver Physiology, 294*(1), G208–G216. doi:10.1152/ajpgi.00398.2007

15. Liu, W., Chen, Y., Golan, M. A., Annunziata, M. L., Du, J., Dougherty, U., . . . Li, Y. C. (2013). Intestinal epithelial vitamin D receptor signaling inhibits experimental colitis. *Journal of Clinical Investigation, 123*(9), 3,983–3,996. doi:10.1172/JCI65842

16. Kriebitzsch, C., Verlinden, L., Eelen, G., Tan, B. K., Van Camp, M., Bouillon, R., & Verstuyf, A. (2009). The impact of 1,25(OH)2D3 and its structural analogs on gene expression in cancer cells - A microarray approach. *Anticancer Research, 29*(9), 3,471–3,483. Retrieved from http://ar.iiarjournals.org/content/29/9/3471.long

17. Vanoirbeek, E., Krishnan, A. V., Eelen, I. G., Verlinden, L., Bouillon, R., Feldman, D., & Verstuyf, A. (2011). The anti-cancer and anti-inflammatory actions of 1,25(OH)2D3. *Best Practice & Research Clinical Endocrinology & Metabolism, 25*(4): 593–604. doi:10.1016/j.beem.2011.05.001

18. Adida, C., Crotty, P. L., McGrath, J., Berrebi, D., Diebold, J., & Altieri, D. C. (1998). Developmentally regulated expression of the novel cancer anti-apoptosis gene survivin in human and mouse differentiation. *American Journal of Pathology, 152*(1), 43–49. Retrieved from http://www.ncbi.nlm.nih.gov/pubmed/9422522

19. Staff. (2014, July 22). Pathogenic connection between autoim-mune disorders, cancer found. *ScienceDaily.* [Web log message]. Retrieved from http://www.sciencedaily.com/releases/2014/07/140722142411.htm

20. Kusner, L. L., Ciesielski, M. J., Marx, A., Kaminski, H. J., & Fenstermaker, R. A. (2014). Survivin as a potential mediator to support autoreactive cell survival in myasthenia gravis: A human and animal model study. *PLoS ONE, 9*(7), e102231. doi:10.1371/journal.pone.0102231

21. Patel, K., & Taub, D. D. (2009). Role of neuropeptides, hormones, and growth factors in regulating thymopoiesis in middle to old age. *F1000 Biology Reports, 1*(1), 42. doi:10.3410/B1-42

22. Hidalgo, A. A., Deeb, K. K., Pike, J. W., Johnson, C. S., & Trump, D. L. (2011). Dexamethasone enhances 1α,25-dihydroxyvitamin D3 effects by increasing vitamin D receptor transcription. *The Journal of Biological Chemistry, 286*, 36,228–36,237. doi:10.1074/jbc.M111.244061

23. Staff. (2014). Drugs that deplete: Vitamin D. *University of Maryland Medical Center.* [Web log message]. Retrieved from https://umm.edu/health/medical/altmed/supplement-depletion-links/drugs-that-deplete-vitamin-d

24. Bokarewa, M., Lindblad, S., Bokarew, D & Tarkowski, A. (2005). Balance between survivin, a key member of the apoptosis inhibitor family, and its specific antibodies determines erosivity in rheumatoid arthritis. *Arthritis Research & Therapy, 7*, R349–R358. doi:10.1186/ar1498

25. Hebb, A. L., Moore, C. S., Bhan, V., Campbell, T., Fisk, J. D., Robertson, H. A., . . . Robertson, G. S. (2008). Expression of the

inhibitor of apoptosis protein family in multiple sclerosis reveals a potential immunomodulatory role during autoimmune medi-ated demyelination. *Multiple Sclerosis Journal, 14*, 577–594. doi:10.1177/1352458507087468

26. Li, F., Ling, X., Huang, H., Brattain, L., Apontes, P., Wu, J., . . . Br6attain, M. G. (2004). Differential regulation of survivin ex-pression and apoptosis by vitamin D3 compounds in two iso-genic MCF-7 breast cancer cell sublines. *Oncogene, 24*, 1,385–1,395. doi:10.1038/sj.onc.1208330

27. Wang, W-L. W., Chatterjee, N.,Chittur, S. V., Welsh, J. E., & Tenniswood, M. P. (2011). Effects of 1α,25 dihydroxyvitamin D3 and testosterone on miRNA and mRNA expression in LNCaP cells. *Molecular Cancer, 10*, 58. doi:10.1186/1476-4598-10-58

28. Zhong, W., Gu, B., Gu, Y., Groome, L. J., Sun. J., & Wang, Y. (2014). Activation of vitamin D receptor promotes VEGF and CuZn-SOD expression in endothelial cells. *The Journal of Steroid Biochemistry and Molecular Biology 140*, 56-62. doi:10.1016/j.jsbmb.2013.11.017

Chapter 6

Should We Be Taking a Vitamin D Supplement?

Should We Be Taking a Vitamin D Supplement?

1. How do I get the vitamin D my body needs? (n.d.) *Vitamin D Council.* Retrieved from http://www.vitamindcouncil.org/about-vitamin-d/how-do-i-get-the-vitamin-d-my-body-needs/

2. Holick, M. F., Binkley, N. C., Bischoff-Ferrari, H. A., Gordon, C. M., Hanley, D. A., Heaney, R. P., . . . Weaver, C. M. (2011). Evaluation, treatment, and prevention of vitamin D deficiency: An Endocrine Society clinical practice guideline. *Journal of Clinical Endocrinology & Metabolism, 96*(7), 1,911–1,930. Retrieved from https://www.endocrine.org/~/media/endosociety/Files/Publications/Clinical%20Practice%20Guidelines/FINAL-Standalone-Vitamin-D-Guideline.pdf

3. Vitamin D Overdose. (2013, September 7). *News-Medical.Net.* [Web log message]. Retrieved from http://www.news-medical.net/health/Vitamin-D-Overdose.aspx

4. McMahon, G. (2010, December 3). Hypercalcemia. *Now@NWJM, New England Journal of Medicine.* [Web log message] Retrieved from http://blogs.nejm.org/now/index.php/hypercalcemia/2010/12/03/

5. Moyad, M. A. (2009). Vitamin D: A Rapid Review. *Dermatology Nursing, 21*(1), 8. Retrieved from http://www.medscape.com/viewarticle/589256_8

6. Garland, C. F., and Baggerly, C. A. (2010). Disease Incidence Prevention by Serum 25(OH)D Level. *GrassrootsHealth..* Retrieved from

Vitamin D Deficiency and Autoimmune Disease

http://www.grassrootshealth.net/media/download/disease_inci-
dence_prev_chart_032310.pdf

About the Author

Wayne Persky BSME

Wayne Persky was born, grew up, and currently lives in Central Texas. He is a graduate of the University of Texas at Austin, College of Engineering, with postgraduate studies in mechanical engineering, mathematics, and computer science. He has teaching experience in engineering, and business experience in farming and agribusiness.

After the onset of severe digestive system and general health problems in the late 1990s, he went through extensive clinical testing, but the GI specialist failed to take biopsies during a colonoscopy exam, and even failed to test for celiac disease. Afterward, not surprisingly, he was told by his gastroenterologist that there was nothing wrong with him.

Unable to find a medical solution, he was forced to use his research skills to discover innovative ways to resolve his health issues. After extensive study, he identified the likely source of the problem as food sensitivities.

It took a year and a half of avoiding all traces of gluten, plus trial and error experimentation with other foods, and careful record-keeping, to track down all of the food issues. But once he eliminated all of them from his diet, he got his life back. He currently administrates an online microscopic colitis discussion and support board, while continuing to research medical issues that are not adequately addressed by mainstream medicine.

Contact Details:
Wayne Persky can be contacted at:
Persky Farms
19242 Darrs Creek Rd
Bartlett, TX 76511
USA

Tel: 1(254)718-1125
Tel: 1(254)527-3682

Email: wayne@perskyfarms.com

For information and support regarding microscopic colitis, visit:
http://www.perskyfarms.com/phpBB2/index.php

Alphabetical Index

Vitamin D Deficiency and Autoimmune Disease

www.ingramcontent.com/pod-product-compliance
Lightning Source LLC
Chambersburg PA
CBHW050734030426

42336CB00012B/1555

9781732822030